Luciana Avedon's BODY BOOK

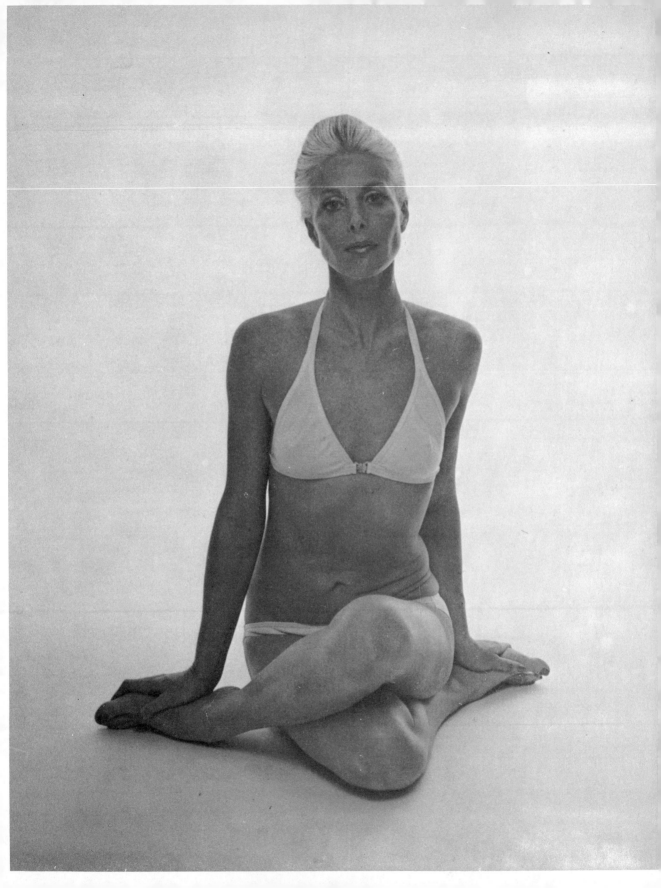

Luciana Avedon's BODY BOOK

by Luciana Avedon and Jeanne Molli
Photographs by Skrebneski

M. EVANS AND CO., INC.   New York, N.Y. 10017

M. Evans and Company titles are distributed in the United States by the
J. B. Lippincott Company, East Washington Square, Philadelphia, Pa. 19105;
and in Canada by McClelland & Stewart Ltd., 25 Hollinger Road, Toronto M4B 3G2,
Ontario

Library of Congress Cataloging in Publication Data

Avedon, Luciana.
    Luciana Avedon's Body book.

    1. Reducing exercises.   2. Exercise for women.
I. Molli, Jeanne, joint author.   II. Title.
III. Title: Body book.
RA781.6.A93   613.7′1′023042   76-15189
ISBN 0-87131-211-5

Designed by Joel Schick

Manufactured in the United States of America

9 8 7 6 5 4 3 2 1

Luciana Avedon's BODY BOOK

Introduction

There will always be glamorous women who declare they do nothing special to maintain their trim, attractive bodies: a zest for living is what keeps you young, they proclaim. I do not envy them; I just don't believe a word they say.

After you're twenty-five, to keep the body beautiful you start fighting the force of gravity, and by the time you're forty, either you take active care of yourself or you are on the ragged edge.

Nowadays no one has the time to spend hours in self-pampering: whether it's good riddance or sad, the overindulged odalisque is dead. (She got too fat and probably drowned in cellulite.) I might add that harem pants flattered big bottoms; modern pants do not. The odalisque never wore bikinis, much less went topless on the beach—in fact, her body never went public. Our bodies do, and that makes all the difference. Busy as we are, though, it is too embarrassing not to stay in shape. Yet if only there were a shortcut: some direct, easy way to get rid of the eyesore and go on with business and pleasure as usual . . .

There is, and it is what I propose. Too bad it is not painless and passive—that is what we would all prefer—but I have gone that route and found it a dead end. To my regret, massage and slimming machines, like miracle diets, get you nowhere in the long run. To stay in shape, you have to decide once and for all that *you* are in control.

Actually, I am convinced more women would exercise if they thought the regimen would work, and I must say that most exercise programs don't produce the desired results. You waste too much effort warming up and flexing muscles that are used enough just getting through the day. Group classes, in particular, are a waste because, to suit all, they suit none. You pay money, and at the end still have the blight that sent you to the class in the first place.

My exercises are a beauty drill for busy people. I don't believe in warm-ups. Unless you are terribly out of condition (when you may need to diet as well), my advice is to concentrate first on improving the part of your body that bothers you aesthetically. A more comprehensive, though always selective, approach can wait, as can preventive measures, much as I believe in them. At my age, I never take anything for granted.

Let's say, to give an example, that you are obsessed by your stomach bulge. Other people may not notice it, but you do, and you're tired of wearing camouflage clothes. Why blur the issue with skipping rope, arm circles, flutter kicks, and rhythmics? Start with one of my exercises for the abdominal muscles. If it seems tough and you have to go slowly for a while, don't let that put you off. When you can increase the count without pauses in between, add another abdominal exercise, then a third. Each one demands a change in exertion. At the same time, become conscious of your posture: hold your stomach drawn up and in.

By the end of a month, the results should be so gratifying that you may want to attack the other areas that also need to be firmed, the ones you don't mind quite as much.

By your starting with the worst problem and seeing that you can successfully cope with it, the others will be easier to handle. Gradually, you will develop the minimum routine, that suits you, personally.

Needless to say, if a bulging stomach is your first concern, it is probably the weak spot you will always have to work on most. Count yourself lucky if that is all you have to worry about. Usually, years of benign neglect take their toll in more ways than one—though I did not choose the example at random. Most women tend to fall apart from the waist down, whether it starts at the stomach, behind, or thighs. We are all sisters at bottom. I know that unless I exercise to prevent it, I am faced with a chronic listing below the belt. Thighs, behind, and abdomen—the latter particularly, if you have had children—constitute the classic combat zones.

Two other areas are also strategic. Whether your breasts are large or small, your pectorals need exercise; and, with age, so does the under part of your upper arm. I call it the applause muscle, because it is the one that flaps in the breeze when you clap. Flabby upper arms are so prevalent that, as *Esquire* put it in an issue devoted to aging, nice old ladies wear sleeves.

My own minimal beauty workout, as illustrated, covers all these parts of the body. Alternate or supplementary exercises are grouped according to the muscles involved. I have also included exercises and stretches for the waistline, neck, and general flexibility. A rigid body, even with good muscle tone, is not very sexy—and even if you are going to bed alone, you will sleep better with the kinks pulled out.

How much you do, and how often, depends on the shape you are in and the standards you set for yourself. Do you really want your best body, or are you content to let it slide a bit as long as you stop the major erosion? Are you active in sports? Do you walk a lot? Is your posture correct? Have you started to exercise as a preventive measure, or because you feel you already look flabby?

Whatever your category, do your program regularly. That means every day—at least in the beginning—and more or less for life. It's like brushing your teeth or taking the garbage out. Once you have learned the exercises for the body areas that concern you, you can put this book on the shelf, to be consulted when new problems arise—but if you shelve exercising as well, it is your body that gathers dust.

For general fitness, 10 minutes' exercise a day keeps you in better condition than less frequent longer sessions, and it's easier to fit into your schedule. Twenty minutes would be better, but let's be realistic: you can always find 10 minutes. One day, for example, you concentrate on abdominals and pectorals, plus a stretch; the next day, you emphasize the legs and upper arm.

For beauty, your mirror is your best monitor. Obviously you must work longer and harder to correct major defects than for figure maintenance, but never underestimate the importance of a steady, constant routine. Age is a prime factor. To have a beautiful body after forty, you have to become an exercise addict. In fact, if you have reached that age in delectable shape you must be already hooked—aware of how you move and what you eat (the good fortune of genes goes so far and no more).

I started to exercise in my mid-twenties and have never stopped. You may be prompted later, perhaps because of some change in your life, but even if you emerge as a late-summer butterfly or as a merry widow, if your beauty motivation is strong enough you will find the grit to pull yourself together. Past forty, better count on 20 minutes a day.

I really think that vanity—call it ego or self-respect—is the key. Were it only for my health, without visible results, I doubt I would stick it out. After all, lots of people whose only exercise is running away from it live to a ripe old age. Were it just for my health, I could try high colonics. (As a matter of fact, I have, and I don't recommend it.)

Portrait of an Exercise Addict

Every afternoon, rain or shine, I am on the floor, back flat as if it were glued to the surface, arms at my sides, one knee bent with foot on the floor, and my other leg with ankle weights, up-down, up-down to a count of 55.

My routine varies little. Rarely does anyone keep me company, and there is none of the fun of sports: sparkling sea, glistening slope, call of the hunt, whack of the ball. Just me, as naked as possible, and my mirror alone in a room keeping score together. Up-down. Up-down.

The nakedness allows for freedom of movement. The weights give maximum effect without my having to repeat the same movement too many times. The mirror acts as a control for both correctness of position and incorrectness of shape: watch that upper arm . . . give that left buttock more of a workout today.

There comes a point when I even enjoy the routine (apart from the pleasure of feeling self-righteous). The repetition, the drone of the count, watching the same, familiar muscles tense and relax—were it not so monotonous, would it have such a reassuring effect, I wonder? For 20 minutes, I think only of my body. What is good for my thighs is good for the world.

In this golden switch of mood, it briefly seems that I want my exercise fix. Without it, how could I stay in touch with myself? How could I live without it? . . .

I know better, of course. By the time I have reached the last exercise of the day, I heave a sigh of relief. As for the next session, February 30 would be soon enough.

Unlike watching the way you eat (after a while, you begin to prefer a balanced diet), exercise is non-habit-forming. Its highs are not the kind that make you feel you cannot wait to turn on again, and the temptation to let it slide does not decrease with practice. Even after years of doing calisthenics, I have not found a way to psych myself into it. I am glad each time that I have done them, I miss the lift that regular exercise gives when circumstance prevents it, but I don't look forward to working out. None of that Girl Scout fervor for me.

My attitude is more realistic than inspirational. Rather than kid yourself, admit that exercise is a bore—and get on with it just the same. You know why you're exercising, and so do I. It gives you direct, intimate satisfaction, no matter what else you accomplish, to have a beautiful body. Particularly when you are not eighteen anymore, it is nice, very nice, to catch a glimpse of yourself and be able to say, "For an old girl, I'm in good shape." That is why you exercise.

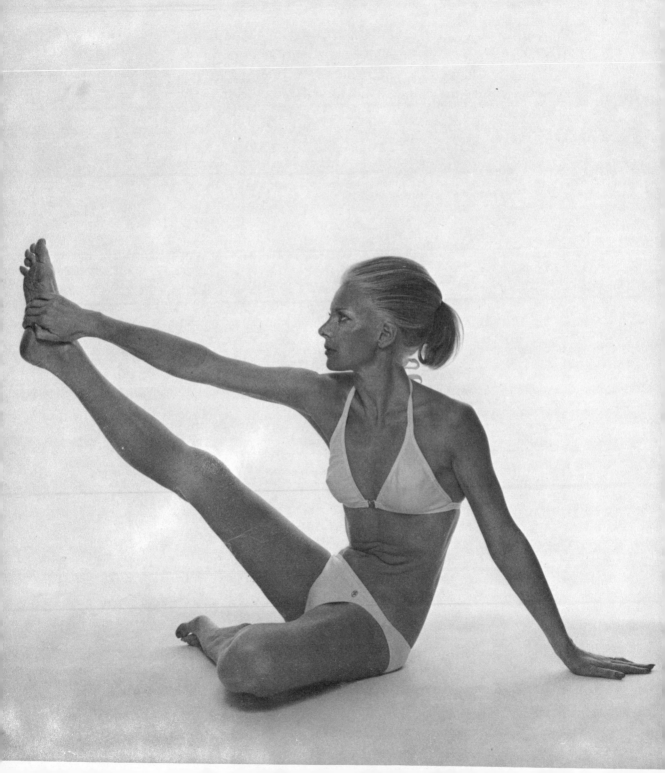

Answering Your Questions on Exercise

How Fast Will I Get Results with Your Exercise Program?

It depends on the shape you are in to begin with: incipient erosion or landslide. With only one trouble spot to correct, theoretically you should get results much quicker, but then again, if it has been a lifelong problem, the "spot" may be more tenacious than general lack of muscle tone can be.

How hard are you prepared to work and what is your goal? Be very realistic. The first spurt of determination should carry you through for a month, exercising 20 minutes a day. Once you begin to notice the difference—and you will before the month is up—enthusiasm will keep you going a little longer, particularly when racing against bikini time. Then it gets tough.

Beauties, like athletes, are in training for life, or at least for as long as they want to play the game. Quick results from concentrated exercise are easy; it is maintenance that is hard. Once you have pulled yourself together and enjoyed the compliments, it is up to you to decide whether to stay in peak form—and why settle for less?—or simply keep trim with a few figure defects. In the latter case, you continue doing the basic program either in 20-minute biweekly sessions or in daily 10-minute segments: Monday it's upper and outer thighs and abdominals; Tuesday it's back and inner thighs and pectorals. . . . Doing less on a regular basis is better than the sporadic big push.

The minimal beauty workout will make you feel healthier and keep you looking pretty snappy. In other words, you may not get top billing, but you will still be right up there on stage.

If you want to star, you have to do more. You know it; I know it. You have to run the full gamut every day.

Should I Exercise Alone?

It is not obligatory, and if you prefer to work out with someone else, go ahead. Some people find it easier to discipline themselves with a friend to keep them company. It is harder to find an excuse to put off exercising if you have made an appointment to work out with someone; and it is also harder to skip an exercise or do only 20 instead of 40 repeats if you don't want to lose face with your friend. Choose someone who lives with you or nearby, so you don't spend more time getting back and forth than actually doing the work.

On a daily basis, I find that exercising alone is more practical for several reasons. Although I try to exercise at a regular time, some days are busier than others. With no one else to think about, I have leeway and can start at six instead of five o'clock, if it suits me better. Alone, I do not waste time gossiping, am finished with my routine in 20 minutes, and have worked intensively, which is more effective than stringing it out with pauses to chat. Even worse, your friend may be a groaner—exercising is bad enough without having to listen to someone moan about it. So if you really want company, put on a record.

Do You Recommend Telling One's Husband?

It all depends on the husband. If he is the kind who teases or says he likes you the way you are when you know you need to shape up, I would not mention it. I would just go ahead, then see if he notices the results. (He should.) After all, if he walks in unexpectedly and catches you in the act, you won't be charged *in flagrante delicto*. When you are married, it is almost impossible to be a closet dieter, because you eat at least one meal together, but exercise can be done at any hour, and in private.

What about Husband and Wife
Working Out Together?

I don't recommend it. Your strengths and needs vary too much. Men tend to fall apart around the waist, and women from there on down. You could do stretches and abdominals together, as well as upper arms and pectorals. (Double the weights for him.) Still, unless you are exceptions to the rule, you need different routines. The approach that is right for you is useless for him.

Can I Exercise in Front of My Husband?

Provided he does not distract you, there is no reason not to exercise in front of any man. It is not a good idea to talk while you exercise, because while you are talking you may lose count, do only 25 repeats on one side instead of 35, and wind up with lopsided thighs.

How Do You Measure Results?

Take your measurements before you start and then one month later. By then you may not bother because you will have seen and felt yourself shrink: your clothes will seem looser around the waist and over the bottom and thighs. Unless you are dieting at the same time, weighing yourself is no criterion. You may not weigh less; in fact, you may weigh a little bit more because you have more muscle. It is the tightening that counts—the loss of sag and bulges and bumps. You can even wear pants without looking like a duck from behind!

What Time of Day Is Best?

Any time, depending on your schedule and your metabolism. For example, I feel great in the morning; I wake up, do a few stretches, and am raring to go. So I prefer to work out in the late afternoon or early evening, the times when I need a break, and exercise revives more than a nap. Early morning, before lunch, or late at night may suit you better. It does not matter, as long as you fix on a time and make it a habit. Forget the idea of exercising at random, whenever you have a free moment, because in that case the free moment never comes. The trick is to make exercise an integral part of your day.

What Sort of Surroundings Do you Recommend?

The ideal setup would be a private gym at home with an exercise bar, rings, ropes, and a masseur on call. I have never had the luxury, and had I waited for it, I hate to think what shape I would be in today. One reason I used to work out at gyms was that I believed the atmosphere and array of equipment were crucial for good results.

Little by little, I realized that results depend on the person, not the place.

Any area in the house that has enough room for a full-length mirror and space in front of it will do. If possible, your equipment (weights, inner tube, umbrella, and mat, if needed) should be stored there, ready and waiting for use. You can choose the bedroom, bathroom, cellar, attic, or hall. If exercise is part of your daily life, you should devote living space to it. Psychologically, this is important, especially in the beginning, because the physical presence of an exercise corner itself reminds you to do your routine.

Once the habit is ingrained, you will find you can do my exercises anywhere: in a hotel room, in the garden when the weather is nice, on the beach. . . .

What Clothes Should I Wear?

The fewer garments, the better. Unlike with sports or gym work, you do not need a special outfit to exercise at home. Striptease is more like it. I prefer working in the nude or near-nude so I can watch what my muscles are doing. A bikini or panties are sufficient. If the room where you exercise is cold, any comfortable, nonconstricting clothes will do—a leotard, for example—as long as they are figure-revealing. After all, the only reason you are going through this whole routine is to make your body look sensational. At first, seeing all your figure faults will spur you on. Later it is very pleasant to note how well you're shaping up.

How Much Equipment Do I Need?

Very little, and in a pinch just bring your body along. The point of no return in gadgetry for home exercise is quickly reached. (So is the point of hysterics with conveyor-belt massagers and wired pads to attach to yourself. It is not true you can just relax and read a book—they tickle!) We have all bought enough let-it-work-for-you exercise gear to know that it usually winds up in a closet, working for no one. Unless you have enough space to set up a home gymnasium, the idea of dragging out the equipment each time is totally discouraging.

I have used cubes to illustrate certain exercises in this book, but I do not own any. The contrast of cubic shape and my own made a clearer illustration. Generally I use any furniture of the proper height that is available: a cane chest of drawers in New York, a bathroom sink in Rome, a dressing table in St. Moritz. . . . Even when one is traveling, there is always something serviceable: a desk in a Denver hotel, the side of the bed in a Kansas City motel. . . .

As basic equipment, I do recommend some form of weights, an old inner tube, and an umbrella. After years of experimenting with anything new, I have finally realized how little you need, but that "little" does make a difference. Flexible weights to wrap around ankles or wrists or to clutch in your hands cut exercise time by half. They come ready-made; homemade sandbags or lead weights sewed into strips of cloth also do the trick. Five-pound weights are adequate— you can always increase the weight by wrapping two on each ankle as your muscle tone improves.

The inner tube and umbrella are used for upper arm, shoulder, and pectoral development. The resistance they

15

provide increases effectiveness, while saving time. If you have lost your umbrella, a broomstick can substitute.

For working out on tile, wooden, or marble floors, an exercise mat is advisable; with carpeting, it is superfluous. Exercise mats are available in sports departments. You can buy foam rubber and cover it with sturdy, washable material or use a bath mat or a sleeping bag.

Of course, it would be fun to have a trapeze in the living room, and perhaps someday I will. Recently a chinning bar was installed in my bathroom. Like all new toys, it is getting a lot of use, but give it a year and I will see if I use it as much. One gadget with more than novelty value is the "wheel," a small rubber tire with handlebars for an axle. Grasping the handles, you do push-ups with it, if you can; sprawls are more likely in the beginning. (Watch out for your back; but if you go at it gradually, it is a great back strengthener, as well as a builder of pectorals and abdominals.)

Should I Get My Doctor's Approval for Exercise?

This depends on your age and physical condition. My program, though effective aesthetically, is not strenuous. Apart from the easy stretches, many of the exercises are done lying down with specific muscles at work and the rest of the body in repose.

Nonetheless, if you have a health problem other than acne or the seven-year itch, by all means get your doctor's approval. Most M.D.'s know too little about physical culture, one of the best preventive medicines, but they do know if you should abstain or take certain precautions. For example, what is the condition of your back? Whether due to bad posture or fads such as platform heels that throw the body out of line, back problems are no longer confined to the geriatrics ward. Teen-agers have them as well.

Should I Exercise on an Empty Stomach?

The theory is that exercise immediately after eating interferes with digestion, although generations of school kids seem to have survived racing around the playground after lunch. I recommend exercising on an empty stomach, although after a light meal, it won't hurt to shake a leg.

Can I Exercise during Menstruation?

I don't see why not, if you don't suffer from cramps. If, however, your period puts you flat on your back, you can do a few stretches, but you may not feel up to much more. (Meanwhile, I hope you endeavor to find out why such a natural manifestation bothers you so much.)

We have come a long way from the era of Victorian prudery when any physical activity, including sex, was discouraged during menstruation. Today, sex is encouraged. It relieves menstrual cramps, the manuals say, which is not the most exciting reason for it.

Nonetheless, it was not only sex that you were not to indulge in during menstruation: the mayonnaise would curdle, plants would wither at your touch, and heaven only knew what would happen if you went swimming or took a bath. Because I belong to a generation that grew up brainwashed by these notions, I still tend to treat myself gingerly on the first day, more from habit than from any real need. I exercise, but I exercise less. After the first day, it is the full program as usual. As we all know, if you are looking for excuses not to exercise, many come to mind. Every time I am tempted to use menstruation as an excuse, I remember the days when I used to ride and go fox-hunting in season— then my period had no effect on my activites.

Is Your System Too Advanced for Someone Who Has Never Exercised Before?

Unless you have an overweight problem, my advice is to plunge right in while you still have some muscle left. The system is not too advanced as long as you adjust the count to your capabilities and build up gradually. (When you first hit the beach, you do not lie in the sun for hours. The first day you take a little sun to form the base for a tan, then gradually you take more until your skin is acclimatized.) If you have never exercised, do what I do, but do less. Start each exercise with a single weight, not double, and do it 10 times, increasing over the weeks until you reach 40. In the beginning, take time to rest between movements. You may feel disheartened because your level of competence is low, but you are moving in the right direction. Exercise that is so mild it is easy to do is even more discouraging, for the simple reason that you get no results.

Will Exercise Make Me Lose Weight?

The only way to reduce is to eat more sensibly than you do. Exercise may help redistribute the bulk and firm up the flab —women wrestlers are not skimpy—but unless it is combined with a change in diet, you will still carry excess baggage; and the more you carry, the greater the strain on your health as well as your looks. Over the years, regular exercise helps you to maintain your proper weight. It also allows for impromptu splurges; enjoy that chocolate mousse or the snack of cheese and crackers. But the following day it is back to frugality as usual—or welcome to the fat farm.

Is There an Age Limit?

I started exercising regularly in my mid-twenties. Until a few years ago, all I needed—and could manage—was 30 repeats. Happily, my endurance seems to have increased. As you age, you have to work more to keep your body toned. My average now is 40, and there are periods when I am not traveling that I can do 50 to 55.

It is the same familiar litany: the older you are, the more care you have to take if you want to look good. You use more creams, spend more time applying your makeup, keep more regular hours. . . . It is like keeping up an old house: the maintenance never ends; and sometimes I think, let it slowly decay. But I'm fond of old houses, fond of myself, and I intend to preserve what I can.

Past middle age, the count begins to diminish, though not the habit of regular exercise. My mother, for example, began to exercise at age fifty-five. She still continues at seventy and is convinced that the best remedy for her morning back pains is her half hour of calisthenics. Her instructor Enzo Sbarra (with whom I also trained) worked on her mental outlook as well as her physical conditioning. First he broke her of the girdle habit (it is bad for circulation) so that she would use her own muscles for support, and he also convinced her that she had to lose weight. My mother thought she would feel weak and wouldn't survive if she lost even four pounds. She lost fifteen, never felt weak, and is still going strong. Her program now consists mainly of leg exercises for inner, outer, front, and back thigh (which she does with one five-pound weight per ankle); sit-ups for the abdominals; the "applause" muscle lift; and a scissors exercise for pectorals, shoulders, and upper arms. Her average count per exercise is 30 repeats.

If Exercise Makes Me Ache Should I
Wait until the Ache Goes Away
Before Starting Again?

My reaction is to work against the ache: the next day do less
of a movement that hurts, but do it a few times and keep at
it until the ache disappears. Don't worry, it will. Exercises
like mine are not geared for Olympic champions. The ache is
a sign that you have used a muscle that was in need of use—
a muscle you forgot you even had. It is very pleasant to
discover something, even if it screams. You feel very
virtuous about the effort. Of course, you feel even better
after a few days when the muscle no longer aches—so have
a good soak in the tub, rub in some cream, and forget it. One
exception is backache above and beyond minor soreness in
the middle or shoulder-blade region. Don't ever force your
back—or your knees.

Does Exercise Relieve Tension?

It relieves muscular tension—but I am not sure about
psychic strain. (And which comes first?) Doing my exercises
gives one renewed energy: you think you feel exhausted, do
the drill . . . and presto, are back on your feet again. As for
real unwinding, I confess that I have never solved the
problem. I suffer from insomnia, although when I did yoga I
could fall asleep in a wink. I know there are various therapies
for total relaxation that operate on the self-hypnosis
principle. You have to stick with them and set aside time

every day. I would rather spend the half-hour on my body instead. In other words, I have made my choice, and beauty is high on my list of priorities. When I feel too tense, I take a tranquilizer. I don't expect any one discipline, including exercise, to be a panacea. I exercise because it keeps my body in shape; the relief of tension and fatigue is incidental, though welcome, and cannot be guaranteed.

What Do You Think about Running in Place?

I think of comic-strip character Andy Capp trying it out and explaining to Flo she could lose a bit of weight. "You just go faster and faster and stay in the same place."

Flo replies, "I'm already doin' a similar sort of exercise— it's called 'earning a living'!"

Running in place, done long and consistently enough, is good for the heart and lungs and revs up the circulation. My exercises do much the same, with less strain, and eliminate your body bulges as well.

Is Jogging Good for You?

Do you live out of town and have a dog? Then jogging fits into your life-style beautifully. Depending on your condition, you might have to build up gradually, but assuming you give the dog a run every day, jogging becomes a game.

Jogging does not replace other forms of exercise, though, since certain key muscles still need a workout. Regularity and clean air are the keys. I do not advise doing it in spurts after you've been sitting for weeks in the office having french fries for lunch and accumulating a spare tire around your waist. If you jog in the city, you will be inhaling those wonderful exhaust fumes, and only polluting yourself.

Do You Advocate Cycling?

Indeed I do. Not only is it excellent for your thighs, back, behind, and abdominals, it's fun and suitable for people of all ages. Again, it depends where and how you live. In the suburbs, in the country, or on a college campus, you can really use a bike and enjoy it. In most cities, setting aside the high risk of theft, you soon begin to feel that the hunting season is open, and you are the quarry. Get stuck once or twice behind a bus . . . find yourself run to the curb by jockeying taxis . . . and the next day you leave the bike at home. When you decide to use it again, the tires need pumping, the weather is bad: the bike sits and so do you.

Biking, like skating, dancing, table tennis, or bowling, can build muscle tone and sharpen reflexes, provided you do the activity on a regular basis. If you cycle for miles every day, you should be able to skip my leg exercises and concentrate on the muscles that cycling does not affect.

As for those home cycling contraptions, they will end up as towel racks or silent butlers for discarded clothes. One reason I don't recommend them is that you feel like a perfect fool, pedaling up a storm and getting nowhere.

I Swim Every Day, Play Golf and Tennis
Several Times a Week, Ski in the Winter—
Do I Need Other Forms of Exercise?

"You're a better man than I am, Gunga Din"—but where do you ever find the time? If you love swimming enough, it is true you can organize your life to get to an indoor pool most of the year, change, do your 20 lengths in 12 minutes, dry off, change again, and be back to your business in less than an hour, unless the traffic is bad. Will you feel and look better? You bet.

Except for swimming, few sports develop the body harmoniously, which is my principal aim.

If you are more active in sports than I, who confess to being lazy, then perhaps you need little exercise drill: you and your mirror can answer that. My exercises are designed for the nonathletic who still want to stay in shape, and they concentrate on problem zones. In my opinion, you can play golf for years and your inner thighs will still look terrible. My advice is to play all the sports you love for the love of them (or to win), then do home exercises for your figure problems, which will still need attention. When I am in St. Moritz, for example, watching people trudging uphill or lining up for the ski lifts, I can't believe it is really worth it—I can accomplish more in 20 minutes in my room. Then if I take a long hike, it is because I really feel like one, and I relax and enjoy it. That is how sportive I have become!

Isn't Regular Sex Good Exercise?

Sex is sex and exercise is exercise, unless you are a pro and the former leaves you cold. In that case, I suppose you might as well approach it as isometrics.

I would like to think that you enjoy sex more when you are in good condition, but I am not even sure of that. How many men who lose their waistlines also lose their libido? Just because I would not go to bed with them does not mean there are no willing candidates. Fat married women, according to a survey by two Chicago psychologists, not only want more sex than thin ones, they are getting more, too. For staying in shape, don't count on sex, much as I hope it is also part of your day.

Should I Combine Exercise and Diet?

It depends on how much weight you have to lose. If it is ten to twenty pounds (and you're healthy), the two are a perfect match. The diet slims you down to size while calisthenics firm you up.

If you are very overweight, fifty pounds or more, the diet may have to be so rigid in order to get results that you don't have enough energy for exercising. At fat farms, for example, while you fast no workouts are scheduled, only massage and hydrotherapy. On the no-cal level, it is a tour de force just to get through the day.

As your diet grows less spartan (never try anything drastic, by the way, without medical control) and you begin to shrink, it is time to start exercise. You may still be overweight, but unless you start to pull in the slack, you'll wind up in drape shape. You'll like what you see on the scales and hate what you see in the mirror. Age makes a difference, also: younger skin is more elastic, and younger muscles stronger. Nonetheless, whatever your age, your real body, the one you always knew was there, camouflaged by the fat, needs toning in order to do it justice. I know what you are thinking: dieting is hard enough; if I have to exercise as well, I might as well shoot myself. My answer is that unless you exercise, you might as well.

Trying to do my complete thigh routine with double weights on the ankles does not make sense if your leg still weighs ten pounds more than it should. On the other hand, random exercises will not help your figure. I suggest you start with the following:

1. The Underpass (10 to 20 times without weights).
2. The Side Kick (10 to 20 times without weights).
3. Sit-ups (10 times done the easy way with your arms stretched out behind your head to give you more momentum).
4. The Applause Muscle (20 times without weights).
5. The Side Stretch (20 times without weights).
6. The Pectoral Squeeze (20 times).
7. Neck Rolls (20 times).

As you can see, this approach has less for the legs than the basic program I usually recommend. Even if you are very overweight, you will probably start to slim first from the waist up; the hips, bottom, and thighs are the last to yield. You therefore concentrate on toning the upper part of the body so that your throat line, bust, and arms will look pretty as they shrink. The side stretch helps take off spare tires, as do the sit-ups. The thigh exercises cause no strain on the back and give you a smoother line, so you will start to lose that "saddlebag" bulge.

In due course, you can increase the number of repeats and add other exercises in whatever order you prefer, beginning to use weights when you are almost down to size. You have to work on your legs and bottom sooner or later. Leaving them for last is the reverse of what you normally do, but I have seen too many valiant dieting efforts abandoned because where you lose first, you sag . . . and you figure if that is the result, why bother. So when you are very overweight, I advise that you firm up as you slim down.

Is It Risky to Exercise after Plastic Surgery?

I refer here to plastic surgery on breasts, abdomen, buttocks, and upper thighs. (Regarding the latter three, I do not recommend surgery unless a woman is so out of shape after years of neglect that she cannot cope otherwise.) Follow your surgeon's advice, since people react differently to operations. Generally speaking, it is a mistake either to rush into exercise or to think that you will never have to exercise again.

The temptation, once the fat has been removed, is to return to your old habits: hot fudge sundaes, double scotches, and the never-walk-if-you-can-ride syndrome. Instead, you do have to watch your diet and at some point, if you are wise, regain the muscle to maintain your second youth. Why go through the pain of having yourself cut, if you are not prepared to follow through? Ultimately, the real risk may be your failure to exercise, but consult your surgeon.

Do You Exercise when You're on a Vacation?

If I stay in one place for my vacation, I usually exercise more. Last year, during three weeks in St. Moritz, I was up to 55 times per exercise instead of my usual 40. During vacation you have more free time, and in mountain air, more pep. When I'm traveling from place to place, it's not so easy, but I manage to exercise daily whether staying with friends or in hotels. Once you start looking for excuses, you can always find new ones, and that is how you slide. Even when flying, I used to pack my weights and inner tube, figuring I would rather pay overweight than have it on me. Now I have learned to leave them at frequent ports of call so they will be waiting for me (like a sailor's girls).

How about Business Trips?

They are my downfall. I do not mean quick business trips or regular shuttling, when if exercise cannot be fitted in, I just skip a day. It is when a promotion tour takes me to twenty cities in thirty days that I'm tempted to throw in the towel. I do try to exercise at least 10 minutes a day because I know from experience how hard it is to start cold when I get back home. And exercising even on hectic business trips gives one a fantastic pickup.

Can You Turn Plane, Train, or Car Trips to Exercise Advantage?

Personally, when I exercise, I exercise, and when I travel, I travel. With all the last-minute details to attend to, I am usually so exhausted by the time I board the plane that all I want is a glass of champagne and then a nap.

If I wake up feeling cramped, to revive circulation I flex my toes and ankles, do a few neck rolls, or lift my shoulders up to my ears, tense, release, and let them drop down into place. Planes are not built for the Big Stretch. As a rule, I am more concerned with the dehydration problem than with my muscles, and my main exercise is applying cream. One useful tip: flying is the perfect way to diet without pain—the food is so dreadful, I drink water and happily skip all that plastic pie in the sky.

Trains are less confining—one can get up and move about more. But twenty minutes of concentrated effort once I am unpacked and undressed seems to me to accomplish more than attempting to exercise en route.

When driving long distances, I used to stop the car and get out and stretch from time to time. I displaced a rib while skiing years ago, which in turn affected my neck, with the result that prolonged driving gave me terrible back pain. Now I wear a German elasticized belt that crosses behind and hooks to the front. With the belt, I can drive as much as five hundred miles without my back acting up. Normally I do not believe in any sort of artificial support—girdles are death—but in situations of stress, use anything that helps you out.

Isn't Housework Exercise in Itself?

Some housework may also be exercise, but not the kind that keeps you beautiful. Making beds never helped anyone's inner thighs; washing dishes does not firm the behind.

Magazine articles that explain how housework can do marvels for your figure strike me as the ultimate con. It is bad enough to have to clean house and boring enough to exercise. Prolonging both by combining them is strictly for Ms. Masochist. Furthermore, unless you keep the refrigerator door shut, all those pliés, jetés, and pas de deux you do with the mop wind up as extra pounds.

Can I Get Exercise Mileage Out of Office Work?

That is another clay pigeon that should be shot down. Yes, you can do standing push-ups against the file cabinet or lift your legs so they shoot out straight from the seat of your chair (tense, hold, release, and return feet to floor). Or, in the isometrics department, try pressing your outer legs against the inner sides of your desk (again, hold and release). But somehow you always seem to be caught in the act, interrupted by the telephone or by someone walking in.

I do have a few suggestions in the nonexercise category to help keep you in shape:

1. When you sit for hours on the job—and this applies to *all* sedentary occupations—the only way to sit is straight, with your back supported, head up, and abdomen tucked in.

Other positions, which may seem more comfortable, will in the long run cause aches and pains, to say nothing of bulges and spare tires.

A. There is no need to following the finishing school admonishment "Girls, keep your knees together." The acceptance of pants for office and other work eliminates that old obsession with the crotch. Actually, modesty did have some virtues: knees together maintained good body line. You cannot slouch, and the feet either rest evenly on the floor or are side-swept by a demure crossing of the ankles.

B. As long as you keep your back straight, you can do what you want with your legs, but if you want trim thighs watch your posture. For example, when crossing the knees becomes a habit, make sure you change sides. Constant pressure on one thigh makes it heavier than the other.

C. I don't do yoga, so it is not comfortable for me, but sitting in the Easy pose (Sukhasana) or the Perfect pose (Siddhasana) keeps the body free of tension and aligned. These are variations on the simple cross-legged position that any child assumes quite naturally while playing on the floor. The difference is that as you fold in the first leg for the Easy pose, the foot must curve under the thigh near to the groin. The second foot then folds under the first, also at groin level. The knees are splayed almost flat. When sitting on a chair instead of the ground, the lowest part of your back is pressed against the back of the chair, a helpful reminder to keep it straight.

For the Perfect pose, the second leg is folded over the first, with the heel hoisted against the pubic bone. The toes curl in the cleft between thigh and calf, and the knees are splayed flat as usual.

No one I know works in full Lotus (Padmasana), but the other poses, I am assured, are more congenial and attractive than the average office slump. Take care to alternate the leg you put on top.

2. Check that your chair is comfortable, either an adjustable model or one built to make sitting straight easy for you. Is the lighting adequate? Are the desk top–chair seat levels correct? Perhaps a footstool or pillow will solve the problem. When you spend seven to eight hours a day in an office, your work tools are very important. Plants, wall-to-wall carpeting, water fountain, colors approved by the resident psychiatrist, and so on, are all very well, but we are concerned with basics here. The wrong desk or chair are bad for your spine, and what is bad for your spine is bad for the company.

3. Sedentary work, even in optimum conditions, calls for a stretch break now and again. You do not have to lie down or swing about —you can do that at home. The idea is to keep your neck, shoulders, and upper back loose. Tension in this area, as osteopaths can tell you, is a classic writer's and journalist's complaint. To avoid it, try the following:

A. Neck rolls: place chin between collar bones, then roll right touching right jaw to right shoulder, base of the skull to nape of the neck, left jaw to left shoulder, chin between clavicles again. Reverse to the left. Repeat several times. Hear the neckbones crack.

B. Raise arms straight overhead, clasp hands in an arch, pull up and from side to side. Then with hands still clasped, bend left arm until the elbow snuggles against the side of the rib cage and the right forearm embraces the top of the head. Bring arms up straight again. Pull. Bend right arm, etc. Repeat. The upward pull loosens up your shoulder blades. The bent-elbow stretch unkinks all of the back down to the waist.

C. Touch your collarbone with your chin. Hold arms straight out to the back, clasp hands, and pull. Raise chin, drop arms still clasped by the hands. Repeat.

Unlike isometrics, a stretch break is so natural that no one will question what you are doing. One other tip: while working, raise your head from time to time so your jawline does not get pressed into permanent pleats.

What Else Can I Do to Keep in Shape while Going about My Usual Routine?

1. You can breathe correctly—a lot of people don't, or might as well not bother, they use so little air. Shallow breathing has its place in a stalled subway or elevator, or during a smog alert or a traffic jam in a tunnel. In pollution crises, of course, one also reverts to shallow breathing: there's not enough air to go around.

In non-crisis situations, which still make up the bulk of living, the rule is to breathe from the diaphragm. Breathing from the diaphragm, apart from making you feel more resilient, is indispensable for singing and also tends to make your speaking voice more pleasant. Female shrill—those voices that grate on the nerves like fingernails on a blackboard—is often induced by faulty, shallow breathing. Most probably you breathe correctly without knowing it. If in doubt, try the following:

Stretch out on your back. While inhaling, push your stomach and abdomen out as far as possible. Exhale, and slowly pull in your middle until it almost seems to touch your spine. (Repeating this 20 to 40 times a day will strengthen your abdominals.) To make yourself really expand and contract, you have to breathe from your diaphragm. I am not advising that you put your whole stomach and abdomen into breathing all the time—that would be grotesque and a waste of energy—but this exercise is an easy way to become aware of the diaphragm's location and role.

2. Stand relaxed and erect. Don't throw your shoulders back, which is as bad as a round-shouldered stance. Your shoulders should ride easy and down. In a sense, your whole body should fall into place from your shoulders, like a coat on a hanger. Do not stiffen or lock your knees. They should be relaxed, imperceptibly bent, in line with the front of your ankle, not with your heel.

Tuck your bottom in. Sticking it out may look sexier— long legs and jaunty rump are irresistible—but it does not look sexy for long. A jutting behind is open sesame to cellulite and stomach bulge. It also invites back trouble because it throws the back out of line.

Tucking your bottom in makes it easier to hold your stomach and abdomen in place. I don't go along with the idea of keeping them taut all the time. Unless you start to have a pouch, there is no need to tense your abdominals constantly;

just hold them in line. But if you are beginning to bulge, I do recommend that you consciously pull in the slack.

Imagine that you are trying to squeeze through a narrow space—to get to your seat in a crowded movie house, for example. What would you do in such a circumstance? You would pull in your stomach. Do this ten times a day. There is even a built-in bonus; the follow-through automatically makes you lift your bosom—and most bosoms can stand a lift.

3. You can bend properly. When picking up something light from the floor, fold over from the waist with legs straight as if your were touching your toes. You can touch your toes, can't you? To lift a heavy object, do a deep knee bend keeping your back straight. The object is then hugged close to the body so that the thighs as well as the back are called into play.

4. If your work is sedentary—in study, research laboratory, factory, office, studio, or lifeguard's chair—how you sit affects both your beauty and your well-being. You spend so many hours a day warming a seat that how you warm it is vital. (See preceding discussion of exercise mileage in office work.) Whenever you are in a straight-chair situation, you and the chair should synchronize; it's a form of mutual respect.

Assuming your workaday sitting posture is good, your stance correct, and your exercise regular, it seems to me you have earned the right to sink into the upholstery by the end of the day.

You are not entirely off the hook, because there is one catch: when you get up from the cushions, don't flail about like a beached whale: keep your bottom in and make your thighs do the lifting job.

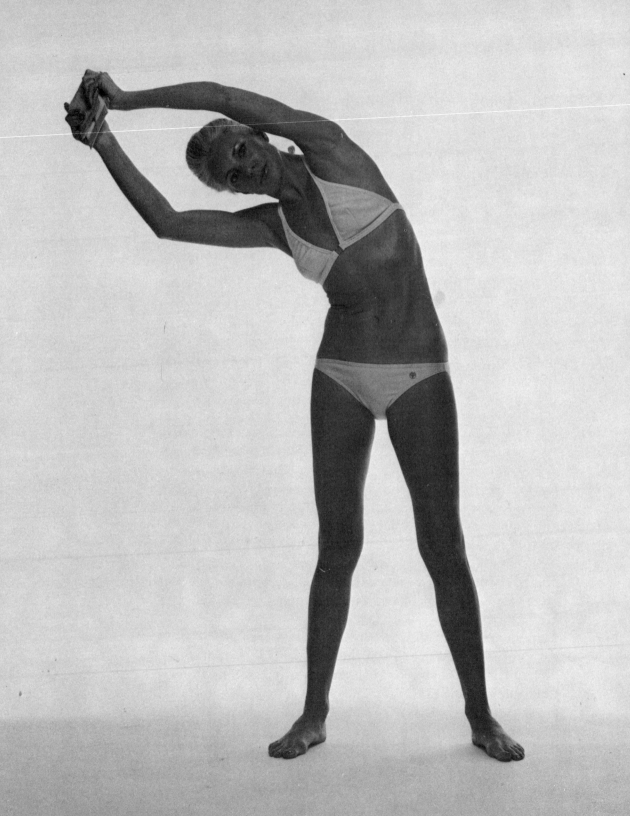

How Can I Tell If I Am in Line?

Stand with feet slightly apart against a wall. Without strain, your heels, calves, bottom, upper back at shoulder-blade level, and head should touch the wall. Don't throw your shoulders back, let them ride easy. There will be a slight gap at the small of the back: that is normal. If you are in line, putting your back up to the wall is an easy check on how to stand properly, not just in bas-relief but also viewed from all sides. On the other hand, if you suffer from lordosis—are sway-backed—you won't get your upper back to the wall.

What Does It Mean to Be Centered?

Any dancer, weight-lifter, or yoga or tai chi practitioner knows that one's strength radiates from the pelvic region. There is no fixed point, because that depends on body build. The fulcrum of a long-legged or high-waisted person will be higher than that of someone with short legs and a long torso. Being centered is having a sense of coordination and equilibrium so that your limbs move freely without throwing you off.

Try standing with your hands on your hips, bend over from the waist, and swing your upper body in the widest possible circle. You will very quickly locate the point that balances the centrifugal force. That is your fulcrum for standing, walking, lifting, and so on. In fact, being centered implies a strong lower back and good abdominal muscles, which many of my exercises are designed to improve.

If I Don't Pass the Line-up Test,
Can I Do Your Exercises?

If you are not subject to backaches, your lordosis is probably mild, and it is about time you started to exercise before it gets worse.

1. When doing exercises for the front of the thigh in supine position (raise leg or legs quickly, lower as slowly as possible), the small of the back is supposed to stay flat on the floor. With lordosis, the small of your back has not dusted the floor for years, so this is out of the question. I have two suggestions:

    A. Do the exercise just the same, but place a small pillow under your back to support it.

    B. While stretched out on the floor, remove the pillow, and before you move on to exercises on your side, relax a minute. Then, starting five times at first, try to make your back hug the surface. Pretty soon it will, and as it does, your stomach will go flatter, and you should get the feeling of proper alignment. Standing properly gives you the same feeling, but it is clear you have not been standing properly or you would not have lordosis. Pressing your back to the floor educates it for proper stance.

2. When doing sit-ups for your abdominal muscles, put a small pillow under your back. Unless your back is strong, you will arch it in order to pull up, and the last thing your hollow back needs is more of the wrong flexibility. Another

38

solution is to avoid the pull-up from the floor. Start sitting up and lower slowly to the floor. This gives your abdominals plenty of work. To return to sitting position, use your hands and arms.

3. Take the inner tube I recommend for other purposes. You don't have to pull it taut; stretch it out with your arms extended over your head. Lower it slowly as far down your back as you can go and raise it up again. This is easy for most people, but if you are hollow-backed with a lower rib cage that protrudes and a stomach that bulges a bit, you will find it hard to do. If you don't have an old inner tube, grasp a length of rope.

Why Don't Your Exercises Emphasize the Back?

If you tuck in your bottom, exercise to keep your abdominals strong, and sit up straight, your back will take care of itself. Actually, most of my exercises do benefit the back although they are designed to combat more visible trouble.

I am not preoccupied by my back, nor are most women. We are more concerned with the state of breasts, belly, and thighs. I know my routine must help the back because mine does not trouble me. The slipped disk I suffered in a car accident no longer bothers me except in conditions of special stress like driving for eight hours straight.

The other reason I do not emphasize the back is that once its condition begins to deteriorate, there is no general remedy. A bad back condition needs the help of a specialist.

As preventive measures, to keep your back supple and strong, the following four exercises are classic:

1. Stand with feet apart, clasping your hands behind your neck. Bend from the waist down 60 degrees from your starting position. Exhale. Raise up. Repeat 20 times. Hold your head straight, your elbows out, and your back straight throughout. For a burlesque variation, hold position at the 60-degree angle, bouncing your bottom in a semi-circle, right, rear, and left. While the simple bend strengthens the middle back, the bounce affects the lumbar region too.

2. Stretch out prone. Clasp hands behind your neck, elbows out, and raise the trunk, keeping your legs on the floor. At first you may need to have someone hold your legs down, or you can anchor your feet underneath a heavy piece of furniture to prevent them from lifting.
The yoga equivalent, called the Cobra, allows you to support the upper part of the body with your arms. The elbows are bent and the hands placed palm downward at chest level. You start by raising the head, stretching the neck outward, then lift the chest and abdomen.

3. The Bow is another yoga movement used to combat central curvature of the spine. Face downward on the floor, you bend your legs at the knees, doubling calves and feet over your behind so you can reach back with your hands to grasp your ankles. Keeping the legs bent at the knees, you force the calves and feet up and back, simultaneously lifting the trunk. The knees may be spread at first, but with practice they should close in. If you can do the Bow, I would

not worry about the condition of your back—it has to be in pretty good shape.

4. Lie on your back, arms on the floor, with palms down. Using your arms as a lever, bring the legs up 60 degrees from the floor, then swing them slowly up and over the head until the toes touch the floor behind it. Reverse to original position. Repeat 10 times. Done quickly, the exercise limbers up the spine; done slowly, it also builds abdominal muscle.

I stress that none of these exercises should be done without medical advice if you have any back trouble.

It is amazing how many bad backs are cured by a good bed. The best has a firm mattress and a low, soft pillow—the weaker the back, the harder the sleeping surface is the rule. Horsehair is ideal, but inexpensive foam rubber will do as long as you put a bed board under it.

Do You Still Advocate
Taking Regular Walks?

I still walk a lot, especially in the country, where the air is clear and you can set a good pace and keep it. Unfortunately, I spend most of my time in the city, where my walks tend to be goal-oriented. While I would not take a bus for twenty blocks, if it is raining, and I have no errands or appointments, I'll choose to stay indoors.

The din, exhaust fumes, crowded downtown pavements, purse-snatchers, and muggers make city walking less and less therapeutic. (Incidentally, I heartily approve closing off downtown areas to cars; that almost restores the faith of lapsed pedestrians.)

The value of walking as a beauty exercise depends, however, on how you walk—and how long. A few blocks' outing with the toddlers, followed by your resting on the park bench while they play, may be exercise for them but not for you. Unless you keep going at a steady pace for at least a half hour, walking is merely a diversion, not exercise. Your lungs will barely notice the difference, and your hips have no time to rejoice.

Some walking, of course, is better than none, and many car-riding Americans have either lost the habit or never acquired it. The technique is simple: your toes are pointed straight, and your legs bend easily at the knees as you shift your weight from one foot to the other. The rest of the body follows the rules of good posture: bottom in, rib cage up, head up, shoulders down, while your arms swing loosely.

What about the Exercise Value of Stairs?

When pregnant with my first child, I lived in a Renaissance walk-up and climbed 102 steps to my apartment. (You bet I counted them.) My post-partum figure was great, and I'm sure those stairs had something to do with it. Needless to say, ever since then I have preferred to take elevators and exercise on the side.

If you live in a three-story house, or a building without an elevator, or vacation in some Mediterranean village perched on a hill with 150 steps between you and the beach, I am sure the constant climbing is good for your legs. It had better be— you have no alternative.

Most people who are not used to climbing feel it first in their calves, but the ache soon goes away. Actually, the thrust of climbing comes from the thighs, which is why it helps firm them. Back straight, hips and bottom under, stomach pulled in, you lead with your thighs—and do not stiffen the knees. Not only does climbing with a bent back look awful, but you'll never make it.

For an exercise plus from stairs, take them on your toes, or if you are in fairly good shape, take the steps two at a time —or on the run. When laden with packages, you should place the whole foot on the tread and go up step by step as usual, with a pause from time to time on landings or mid-stairs. Incidentally, if you are not used to walking upstairs, do not be alarmed if your heart begins to beat faster as you near the top of a long, steep flight. Just take a pause.

What Is the Best Way to Cope with Heavy Parcels and Bags?

Get someone to carry them for you! Unfortunately, these days a good man is hard to find, and that includes redcaps and porters. If you travel a great deal, you might invest in one of those lightweight gadgets that strap on your bag for easy wheeling. I am surprised no one sells them at railroad stations or airports.

The easiest way to distribute weight equally is to carry the load on your back. Foldable backpacks (as opposed to those armored rucksack jobs) are a shopper's and traveler's boon. They leave your hands free, as well as priming your back muscles. I also advocate a return to the old string bags

European housewives used to take to market. Ecologically, they are sound (cutting down on plastic wrappings and bags) and most are designed with straps that are long enough to hang over your shoulder. They expand and when empty can be tucked into a pocket or purse.

Whatever system you use, equal distribution of weight is the key. Most of us tend to favor one side and wind up lopsided as a result. Even when carrying normal paraphernalia—schoolbooks, handbags, or dispatch case—remember to switch sides now and again.

What Can Exercise Do for My Bosom?

Exercise will not make breasts larger or smaller, or lift sag. You need plastic surgery for that, or bras that give the desired illusion.

The breast is a gland, not a muscle, and once it goes, it is gone forever. As a preventive measure, however, you can strengthen the pectoral muscles; even when your breasts have sagged, this will make them look higher and firmer in low-cut dresses or bathing suits. It will make a small bosom look more attractive because it eliminates scrawny, bony décolleté.

In addition to exercise for the pectorals, regular cold showers (use a hand shower if you have one) help firm the breasts. Good posture is also important: shoulders down, stomach in, and rib cage up. Rounded shoulders are an invitation to cave-in, and shoulders back, chest out causes undue strain—save that for your *Playboy* pictures.

I rarely bother with bras because my breasts are small

and my muscles toned. Full breasts benefit by support as long as you do not rely too much on the bra but use your own muscle as well. Find more than one bra design that suits you, and alternate models to avoid constant constriction in the same places.

Do You Recommend Face Exercises?

I have tried many puckering and pursing exercises, sticking out my tongue and aiming for the tip of my nose and my chin. I think they cause more wrinkles than they eliminate. Facials are good for toning and waking up the skin, and standing on your head gives you a temporary lift. So does making love: how smooth the skin becomes—if postcoital depression exists, your face does not know it.

Sometimes I consciously remember to relax my face when I sense I have been frowning. One can and should be aware of tenseness in the forehead and mouth. The neck rolls I preach and practice also aid relaxation, but they will not save the skin of the neck when it wrinkles up like a turkey's, or eradicate smile lines, crow's-feet, and furrowed brow. Silicone micro-injections by an expert will plump up the cheeks; makeup, creaming, and masks can do wonders, but once the face really sags, only plastic surgery will shore it up. (Though dangerous for breasts, liquid silicone for facial sag is feasible because of the very small quantity used. Still, the process takes a year or so and is done a drop at a time so that it will not travel. You don't want to find yourself with dewlaps.)

What Can I Do to Keep My Hands Young and Supple?

Playing the piano is one theory, or becoming a masseuse or typist; all three activities develop flexibility as well as strength. My answer is to cream them. One reason hands tend to age is that they are used, abused, and exposed so much. Maybe they fared better when ladies always wore gloves, never went out in the sun, and always had cooks, maids, and gardeners. Exercise doesn't prevent their aging except that it stimulates circulation. As far as I know, the best thing is plenty of lubrication and wearing something to block out the sun on the beach. (I refer here to "normal" hands. There are exercises for stiff joints and arthritic conditions, which should be prescribed by a therapist on an individual basis.)

Any cream, oil, or lotion will do as long as it is applied often and thoroughly. Keep several bottles within easy reach, by the bed, in the bathroom, in the desk drawer, and in the kitchen. Chemical peeling is often suggested to remove blemishes. The risk, however, is replacing liver spots with scars.

Polish protects your nails to some extent. Adding gelatine to your diet sometimes strengthens them, but adequate calcium intake is their best friend.

What Can I Do to
Have Pretty Feet?

First of all, buy good shoes. Where feet are concerned, no matter what kind you have, quadruple A or E, treat them as though they were a rare treasure. Never fall for the salesman's pitch that if a shoe pinches a bit, it is only a question of breaking it in. That system may have worked when the maid or butler broke in shoes; otherwise, they wreck your feet.

Particularly when you are active or your job requires standing, you cannot afford to save on shoes. Skimp on something else—who needs a nightie, sleep in the nude—but cover your feet with care. Vary your everyday shoes or buy two pairs at a time of your classic favorites. One pair gets downtrodden too fast. (Men make this error more than women.)

Fashion in footwear comes and goes, but I always wear a low or medium heel, and not because I am tall. High heels are strictly for evening (if then), for an obvious simple reason: like wasp waists and balcony bras, high heels are hell on the body. They pitch you off line.

Small feet, thank goodness, are no longer considered chic or erotic—I could never play Cinderella with my pair. As long as they are smooth and strong, who cares? Exercise and diet cannot change the shape of the feet, so one might as well make the best of what one has. The heels and the outside borders and balls of the feet should carry your weight. Unless you are a ballet dancer, walk with your feet placed straight in front of you. Incidentally, it is not true that walking barefoot outdoors enlarges the feet, it only makes them calloused (and dirty).

For tired feet, or to strengthen them:

1. Sit down in a comfortable chair. Clench your toes and relax, extend toes upward, relax again.
2. Using your heels as a lever, raise feet toward the ankle, then push them down as far as they will go.
3. Using your ankles as a pivot, circle to the right, then circle to the left.

For swollen feet: prop them up wherever you can until you get home, then stretch out on the bed with book or TV, swing your legs up from the hips, and rest your feet high against the wall.

The above techniques are simple and can be done in much less time than it takes to prepare and endure one of those depressing footbaths that make you feel you are eighty years old.

The other procedure I recommend is creaming your feet after a shower or bath. Also give the ball and the heel a go with a soapy loofah or pumice stone if walking barefoot has built up calluses. For corns and bunions, or just for an annual checkup, hobble or run to the chiropodist.

My Calves and Ankles Are Heavy—
Do You Suggest Any Special Exercise?

First, how much is body structure and how much is fat? Are your ankles thick but supple, or are they puffy (bad circulation) or painful to the touch (cellulite)? One really cannot change bone structure.

To a certain extent, the ankle rock slims ankles and improves calves. You stand feet slightly apart, hands on hips, knees loose. Rise up on your toes and lower slowly until your heels are back on the floor. Repeat 30 to 40 times and practice daily.

Cycling both slims fat calves and builds up hollow ones. Either hit the road or do the classic home substitute without wheels. Stretch out on your back, arms at your sides. Raise your legs perpendicular to your upper back, supporting them by moving your hands under your rib cage to the back. Raise your pelvis off the floor, resting on your shoulder blades. Then pump away with your legs and cycle upside down.

While improving your calves, this also does wonders for the complexion because the blood rushes to the head and gives your cheeks a healthy glow.

A good masseur ought to be able to whittle off some of your lower-leg heaviness, and proper diet should eliminate puffiness. Also, take rest breaks with your feet propped up high. Bone, however, is bone, and if you have broad ankles (and wrists), you probably also have strong feet (and hands) in proportion.

Of course you do not wear extreme, conspicuous shoes, such as platform shoes, or ankle bracelets, or, if you have heavy legs, short skirts. Fashion is so flexible today that there is no excuse for not wearing what becomes you. Adhere to the longer skirt length your mirror tells you is most flattering, or wear pants, unless you have got a bulky behind —but that, too, can be remedied.

What Can I Do for Legs and Ankles that Swell Up?

For a water-retention problem (and to avoid having one during pregnancy), get your feet up during the course of the day. Proper diet is crucial, but elevating your feet is equally important. Anyone whose job requires prolonged standing needs the Movie Producer's Break: feet on the desk and cigar in the mouth (the cigar is optional). To be more discreet, pull out a desk drawer or use a wastebasket.

In standing-room-only situations, it also helps to flex your thigh and calf muscles from time to time, or just shake a leg. Balance on one foot, and lean against something for balance, and with bent knee and foot raised off the floor, shake your leg out, as if it were a flour bag.

Will Exercise Cure Slackening of the Skin?

When you are young, even with sudden weight loss, your skin springs back easily. In your twenties, your belly after childbirth is wrinkled and soft, but it rarely stays that way if you have the good sense to restore abdominal muscles. If you also had the foresight to cream your belly during pregnancy, stretch marks will be minimal or nonexistent. Older mothers may have to exercise harder to pull in the slack, and it may take longer for them. (By the fifth or sixth baby, don't expect miracles.)

The same holds true for obesity, never a blessed event. The younger you are, the more resilient the skin. Even when you Yo-Yo—putting on twenty or thirty pounds, taking them off, putting them on again—up to a certain age your skin will adjust with few telltale marks. Start to reduce abruptly when middle-aged or older, and not only must you exercise but your skin needs a lot of lubrication during and after dieting. Drop fifty pounds after fifty, and unless you do it gradually, your skin will not snap to attention. Exercise will firm your body and absorb some bagginess, but the skin will probably be looser than it was before.

"But," you protest, "I've never been fat. I wear a size 8 and have kept myself in good condition, except that suddenly I have wrinkles on the knees, and when I bend my arm, the inner elbow fold looks like shriveled leather."

Keep exercising to maintain and build muscle tone; it should arrest the slack. Meanwhile, feed the crepey areas morning and night with cream or oil, massaging with a plucking motion as you apply the grease until it is absorbed. Dry skin does tend to wrinkle with aging, and you notice it first at articulation points. (Bend your foot up sharply, heel on the floor, and you will see horizontal wrinkles just above the ankle bone—a ten-year-old won't have them.)

Any lubricant, ranging from baby oil and pharmaceutical lanolin to twelve-dollar-a-gram famous-name unguents, will do, especially if you change the brand when your skin seems to have lost its appetite for it. The plucking massage should be vigorous—your body can take it. If you get tired of plucking, work it in with a hard brush.

This does not apply to the face or the neck, though slapping in neck cream with an upward movement helps keep that watershed zone from drying out and developing age-revealing lines.

Slackening of the skin affects men as well as women, if that is any consolation. You see middle-aged men on the beach who look trim and cut a very dashing figure . . . until they bend over and it looks as if they are wearing a dress of a thousand pleats.

A few crepey patches may be the price you have to pay for skipping the "fat and forty" dilemma. As long as everything else is up, I would feel pretty proud—and like the Tin Woodsman, I would simply keep my oil can around.

Do You Advocate Massage for Shaping Up or Spot Reducing?

Massage as a supplement to exercise and diet may accelerate the desired results. When your problem is overweight as well as poor body tone, I think you should bring up all the artillery, including saunas or steam baths if you can stand them (I can't). Thalassotherapy and aromatotherapy, both of which involve massage—one with algae and underwater jets; the other with herbal potions—aid circulation and help redistribute weight.

While dieting strenuously, exercise has to be mild, and massage starts pulling in the slack. On the other hand, when you have no weight to lose or it's a question of fifteen to twenty pounds, massage is optional. It does the masseur more good than you, because he or she is the one who is getting the exercise and you are the one who needs it. The exceptions are spot cellulite removal and slimming heavy ankles and calves, for which a combination of massage and exercise is always advisable.

It is very pleasant to be massaged and I would gladly have a masseur on call, were it feasible. The real virtue of massage lies in tension release. Unless you also exercise, you remain the same blob you were before, but you feel so good that for the moment you don't care.

Techniques to choose from range from the lightest touch to such rough treatments as rolfing. (Rather than pamper knots and aches, rolfers are likely to plant their elbow at the stress point, then bear down with all their weight.) While I don't believe you should leave the table black and blue—that does not help circulation—I do subscribe to the vigorous approach. You can get the light touch in the bedroom.

For do-it-yourself massage, walks in the sea with the water waist-level or trout-fishing that gets you wading in streams are excellent. So is a brisk rub-down with a loofah while taking a bath. Use a soaked, soapy loofah, of course; you don't want to draw blood. Rinse off with alternate hot and cold blasts from a hand shower.

Should Children Be Made to Exercise?

If they have an active life, do sports or ballet, play hard outdoors where they can run, skip rope, climb, skate, and ride bikes—they don't need a special exercise program. You do, because you are older and less active physically: it would not occur to you to do handsprings down the road. In city conditions, getting children to sports activities and back requires organization, but as a parent you have to be organized to preserve your sanity.

It is true that some children shun sports and games like the plague. I still would not make them exercise. At most, I would check their posture, as I also would with a sports-minded child. If it is bad, the only solution is to advise them —even to nag them—until it improves.

Provide school-aged children with desks and chairs geared to their size, and make sure they have adequate light wherever they read, even in bed. The same holds for young painters and craftsmen.

If I were you, I would take a sharp look again when your children are past puberty. You have been observing them all along, but girls with growing breasts and heavy thighs should be aided and abetted, and pear-shaped boys overhauled. Teenagers are very sensitive about their bodies, so be diplomatic. Suggestions, not taunts, are welcome. It may be time for spot exercise at home.

Do Your Exercises Build Endurance?

The well-toned legs, strong abdominals, and straight back that my exercises develop should enable you to walk long distances, play sports more energetically, and feel less fatigue in workaday life. On the other hand, my exercises do not make you work up a sweat. They are designed for beauty and harmony rather than strength.

My endurance level under stress is pretty high, but then I also try to lead a regular, disciplined life: I have a balanced diet, smoke little, drink even less, take periodic special cures for my liver, and go to bed early. One theory is that, for fitness, an exercise program should include skipping rope, running in place, or similar intense, fast movement, because of the boost it gives to the cardiovascular system.

I do not do it, but with my program I know I can pass a two-minute step test within the acceptable norm. To do the test, you need a sturdy bench or chair fifteen to eighteen inches in height. Place one foot on the bench, bring the other alongside. Lower first foot to the floor, then the other. Repeat the four-count movement 30 times a minute for 2 minutes. Rest for 2 minutes and take your pulse for 30 seconds, doubling the count to get the per-minute rate.

As pulse rates, even without exertion, vary according to the individual, you or your physician should determine your normal, or average, rate. When you are fit, your heart recovery after vigorous sudden effort levels off more quickly than it does for someone out of condition.

Beauty workouts, including systematic weight lifting for men, do not necessarily prime you for two hours of tennis in the hot sun or enable you to pass an army medical or a marine obstacle course. "Mr. Physique Fails Police Department Physical" has become a classic joke headline.

One advantage of my mild, regular exercise system is that you do not build up fatty tissue should you stop. Muscle-power addicts, who concentrate on building their upper bodies, often build fatty tissue if exercise is discontinued. But apart from this, what do you mean by endurance? I could never do a four-minute mile and might finish last in a 100-yard dash. I don't have the build, much less the life-style, that qualifies for track. My approach makes looking good endure, and it gives staying power for beauty.

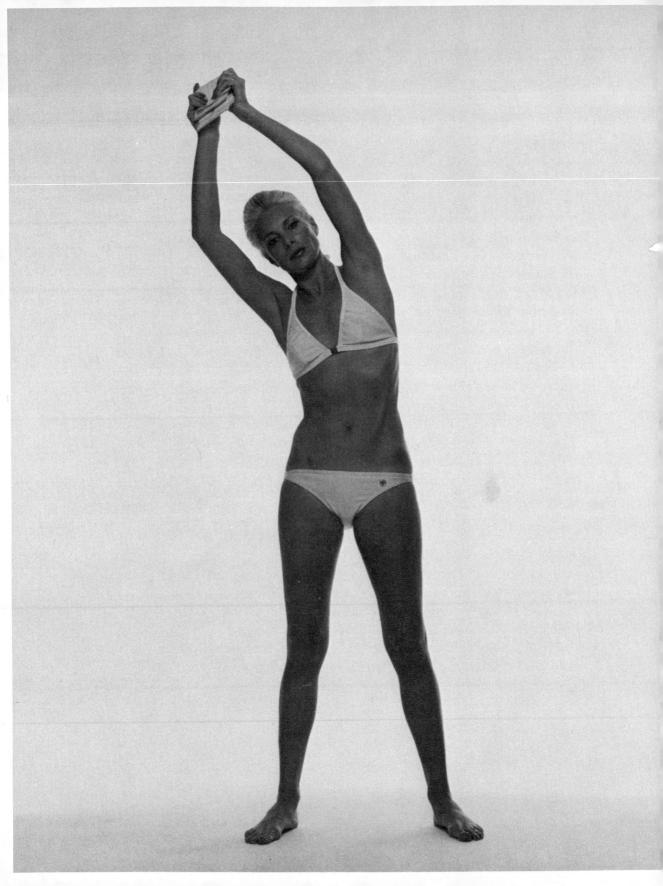

The Minimal Beauty Workout

Let's get down to business. Stretch out on the floor. First problems first. You have not warmed up, but I don't think you need to in a supine position. There is no balance to lose or force of gravity to fight. Stretch out and relax for a minute if you want, legs open and arms folded under your head. Sink into the floor and take a deep breath.

Ready? You are about to exercise your bottom and thighs. By doing this, your buttocks, hips, and back automatically get their share of the action. The rest of you takes it easy.

After the first four exercises, the focus shifts to the abdominal muscles that are so important for health as well as beauty. They support you and are your childbirth muscles; when they go slack they are hard to conceal except in the most voluminous clothing. A pot or sag in the middle makes you look old and tired. Good posture is the key. In addition, any minimal beauty workout should include at least one specific abdominal exercise as cure or preventive measure.

Then the emphasis is above the belt. Your lower half has earned a rest. It can sprawl while you are still on the floor, putting your arms to work. They mostly take care of themselves, but the under part of the upper arm remains a potential "ugly." Like your thighs, this is a zone that normal daily activity does not sufficiently call into play. That is why I include it, giving you also a chance to relax before leaving that welcome mat and getting yourself up on your feet.

In standing position, you do a pectoral tightener and a final stretch that loosens you up, trims your waist, and benefits your upper back. That is it!

Props recommended for the minimal beauty workout are: an old umbrella, flexible weights, and an exercise mat if your floor is not carpeted. For novices at sit-ups, a heavy piece of furniture to anchor your feet under is also advisable. You do not have to use weights in the beginning, but for anyone in reasonably good shape they speed results. (No, they do not give you bulging muscles and popping veins. Even worn double, at ten pounds, they are not heavy enough for that.)

You work at your own speed, resting if need be, between each set of exercises, though I don't suggest resting between repetitions of the same movement. Better to do 5 continuous side kicks than 20 with pauses in between. Eventually you will reach 50 with ease. As you progress, you may wish to add to the program, varying it to emphasize movements designed to correct your personal figure problem. Variety keeps your muscles and interest alert. The alternatives I use are illustrated and explained later in the book.

The Minimal Beauty Workout

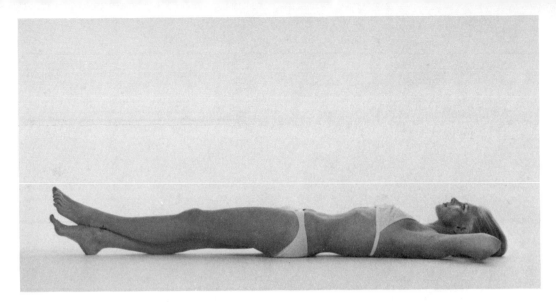

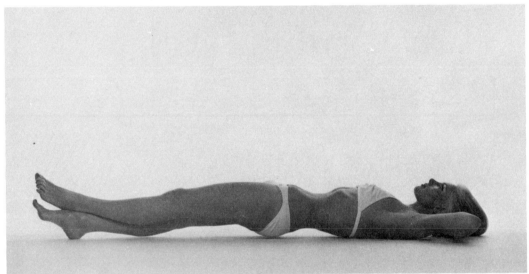

The Clencher

A dual-purpose exercise, the
clencher firms your backside, as
well as the front and back of your
thighs. It looks and is easy to do,
though hard to sustain for a
minimum count of 20 or more.

When 50 becomes a cinch, have
someone sit on your thighs.
 Stretch out, arms under your
head, and cross your left ankle
over your right. Inhale, and
clench and lift your thighs. Hold.

Exhale, and relax and lower your thighs. The stress is on the front of your thighs—that is why it is good for them. However, in hold position, consciously tighten your buttocks so that they, too, derive benefit. I prefer to do 50 with left ankle crossed over on top, then 50 with ankles reversed. If you prefer, you may alternate each time.

For an added fillip, as you exhale and relax to starting position, prolong exhalation an instant longer until you feel your abdomen flatten. Briefly press the arch of your back to the floor. Then inhale, clench, hold as usual. You don't have to do this if it makes you lose momentum.

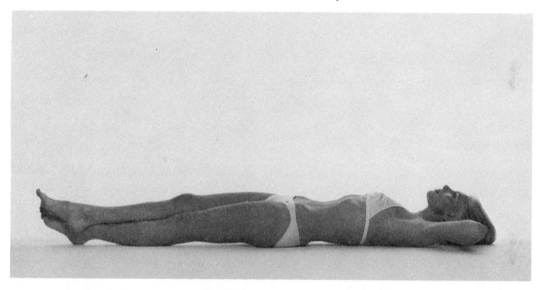

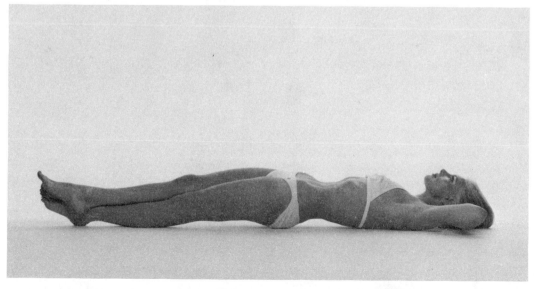

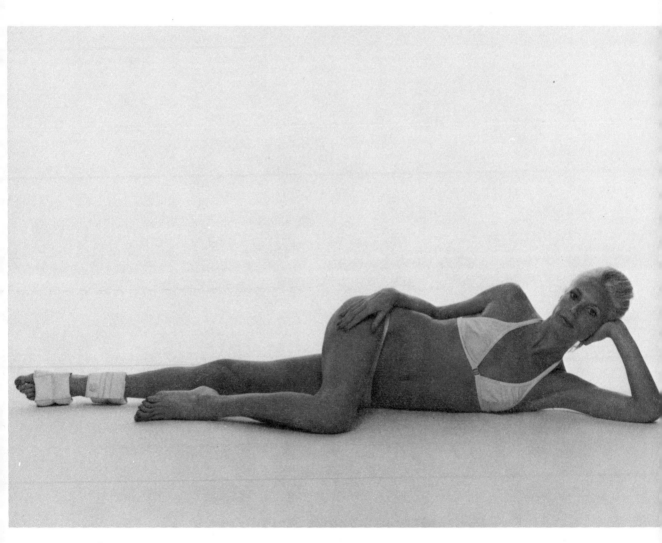

64

The Underpass

This is for tightening inner thighs.

Stretch out on your side, and enjoy looking provocative, one leg crossed over the other and the opposite arm supporting your head. I mention looking provocative because you won't feel it once you get going on this one. You will feel ungainly and awkward because it is not a "natural" movement. Unless you ride, do ballet, or specialize in Tantra sex, you are not used to making this area work. That is why you see so many flabby inner thighs on the beach.

As illustrated, I wear double flexible weights to make it harder for myself. You may prefer to wear none or one, depending on your muscle tone. The important thing is to do the exercise smoothly and properly with or without weights. They can be added later.

Just ordinary walking in a relaxed, lined-up position, instead of locking the knees and teetering in heels that throw you off balance, is the intelligent woman's guide to the maintenance of inner thighs.

Nonetheless, at a certain age, they tend to get flabby. If you can still crush coconuts between your thighs, skip the Underpass. Otherwise, aim for 20, then build up to a count of 50.

Shatter initial languid position by raising underneath leg abruptly and as high as you can. It won't go very high because your other leg, crossed over and at rest, blocks the kick. This is instinctively annoying, but you are not trying out for the Rockettes. Instead, you are rudely awakening a possibly lazy muscle. At whatever height you reach, the point is to sustain the lift briefly.

My non-supportive arm curves over my side with my hand on the hip of my nonworking leg. If it

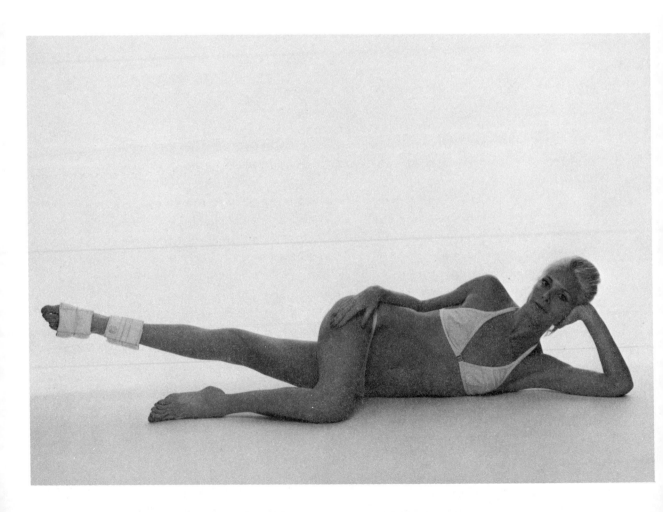

helps, place your hand on the floor, using your arm as a lever. As long as you reactivate the inner thigh, placement of arms is incidental.

Your leg is caught here in center position. Just to raise and lower is rarely enough; in most exercise you need a catch in between. Holding at maximum works the muscle one way; intermediary hold gives it another flex. Try it, and you will sense that the pull is different when you also hold halfway down.

Once you get into stride, your foot should barely touch before you lift up again. Steady, continuous cycle is your goal. Fast up, slow down. Repeat at least 20 times. Roll over and underpass the other leg.

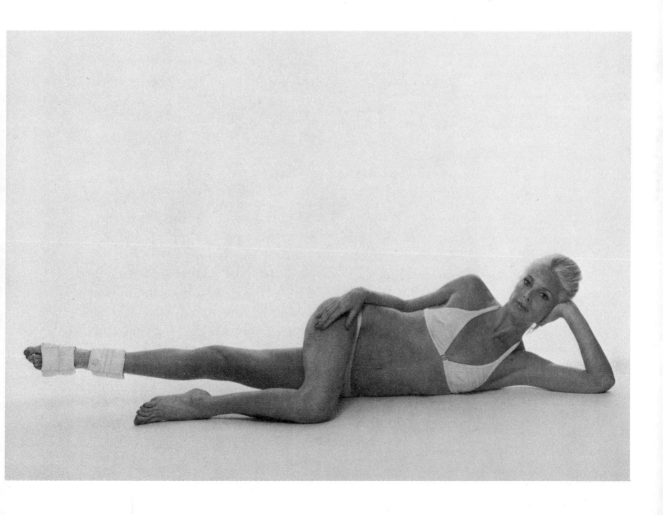

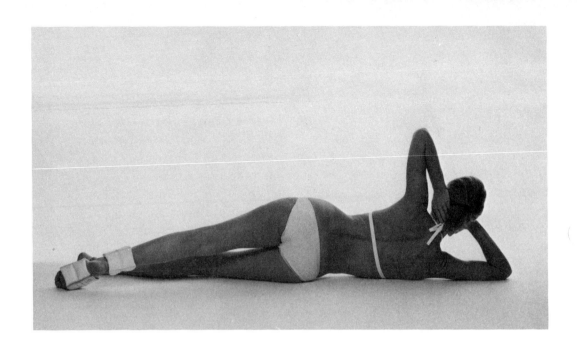

The Side Kick

While still stretched out on your side, you now swing into an exercise that gives you more freedom of movement. Here you can open up, aim for the ceiling, and let go with a series of real kicks. The exercise is easy and highly effective for giving a long, smooth line to your outer thighs. It combats these ghastly saddlebags that bulge, look so terrible in pants, and mean that

ready-to-wear never fits because you are one size on top and a larger size below.

Support your head with one arm. Bend the other and clasp the nape of your neck. Start with the toe of your kicking leg touching the floor just to the back of your leg in repose.

Give a good swift kick as high as you can go, higher than I do if it comes naturally and you still

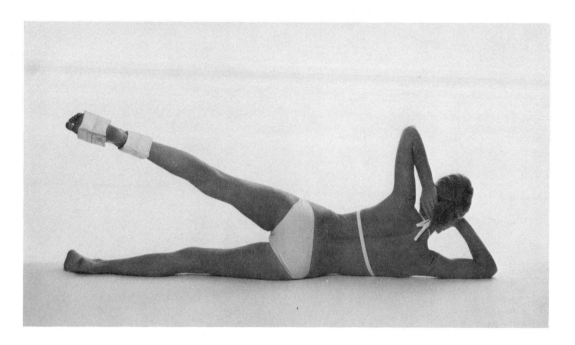

can control the descent. The idea is to exhale at highest point and come down slower with imperceptible holds along the way.

In other words, it is up, down, up, down, up, down without stalling. The continuous movement takes longer on the downbeat.

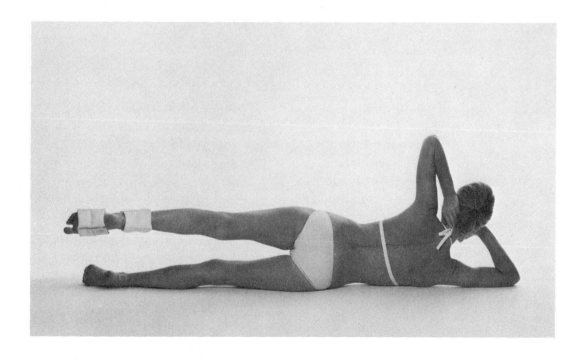

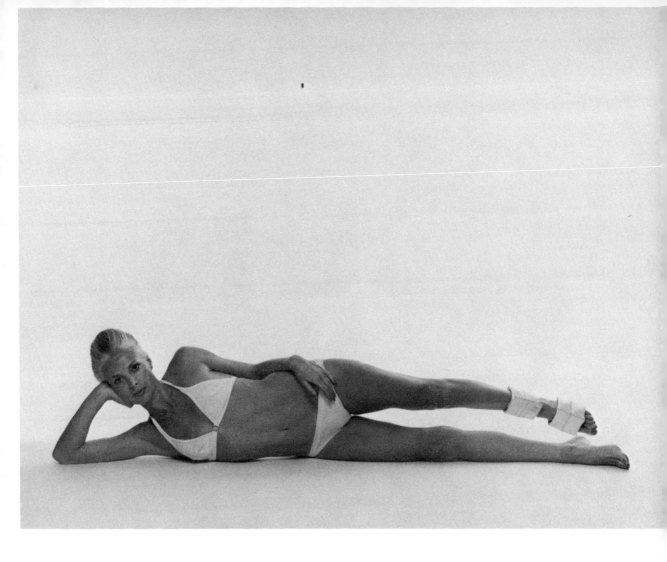

Seen from the front, this is a second logical point to make your muscle feel the weight as you come down. In fact, as you become accustomed to the side kick, this is as far as you should go before swooping up again.

Of course, it is permissible to touch base, though you don't want to land like a sack of potatoes.

Touch, if you must, but make it touch and go.

Note that I have changed arm position again. Here, too, if you prefer, use one arm as a lever, placing the hand on the floor in front of you. That is fine as long as it does not make your kick leg swing to the front—the correct movement is slightly to the rear.

Up you go, and no matter what

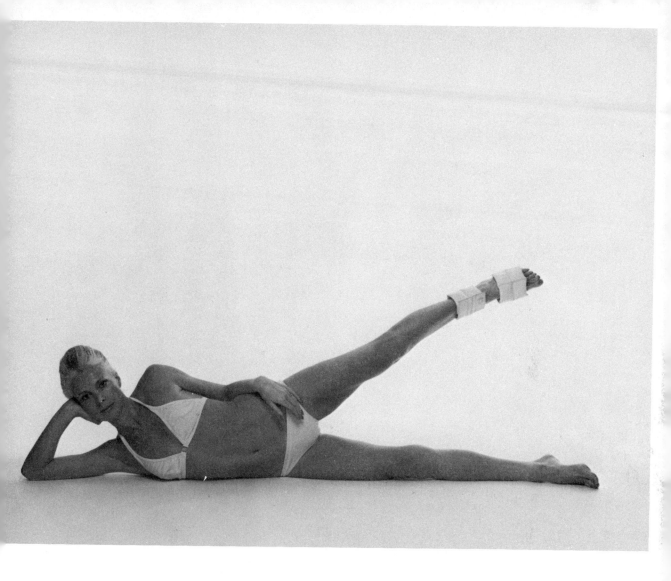

shape your outer thighs are in, there is strong muscle there. A count of 20 without weights is a breeze, and no hardship even when you are carrying extra freight. After all, you are lying down.

When you reach the stage where you want to make it hard for yourself—I find that flat out serves the purpose well enough— you advance to side kicks in vertical position. Hold with one hand any piece of furniture at ballet barre level and do the same exercise while standing up. Just kick out straight and lower gradually. That, too, is easy, so do it like a dancer, with bottom tucked in, feet splayed, and a proper turnout that uses all of the thigh at once.

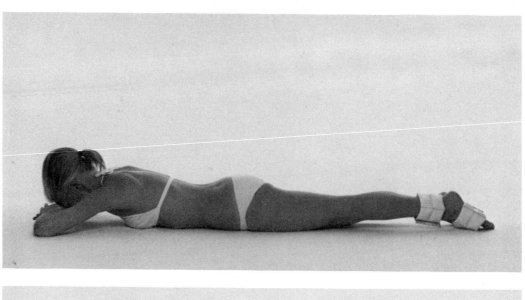

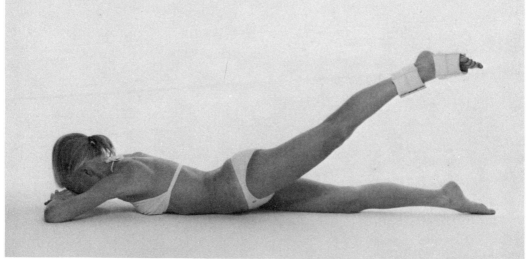

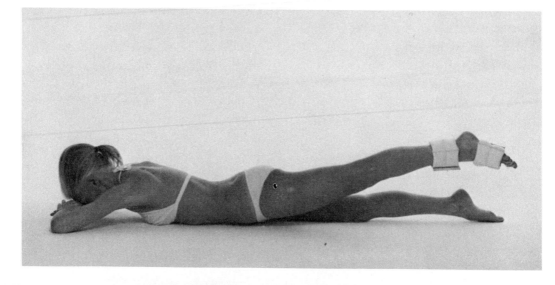

The Back Stroke

For desk workers this is a must because it awakens the part that goes pitted and soft from being sat upon all day: the back of the thighs and the rump. If your idea of sport, once you leave your desk, is to commute by car, watch TV, or play cards, you are a candidate for fanny flab at age twenty-five.

I show the exercise here in its simplest form. In prone position, your head cradled in your arms, you kick up one leg, bring it down slowly, holding at mid-point, touch toe to floor, and kick up again. Lift and lower 20 times, aim for 50. Switch legs and repeat.

When that becomes too easy, try lifting both legs together—

they won't go up as high. Tense at whatever elevation you reach, make a controlled descent, and lift quickly again. You put more stress on your back that way. With a strong back that nonetheless needs limbering, clasp both hands at the nape of your neck or place them on either side of your head for leverage, and while doing the double-leg lift, simultaneously raise your head off the floor.

I don't bother with these refinements and find them distracting. One leg at a time is enough and enables me to concentrate on using my rearguard muscles so totally that I feel the pull up to the hip.

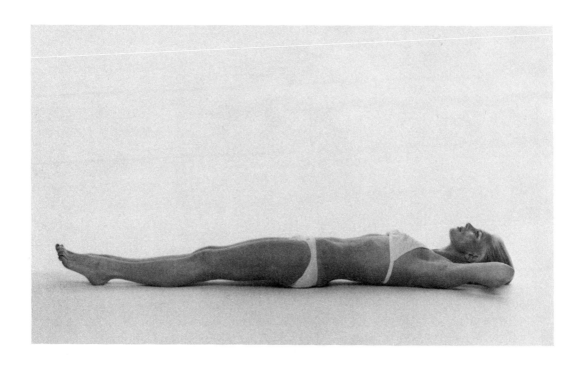

Sit-ups

The standard exercise for
strengthening abdominal muscles
is and will always be the sit-up or
one of its variations. You have
seen it in every exercise manual;
you see it here and I practice it

for the simple reason that it works.

My initial lift, from flat out to
sitting with back straight, is
orthodox procedure. You can
stretch your arms out parallel to
the side of your head to give you

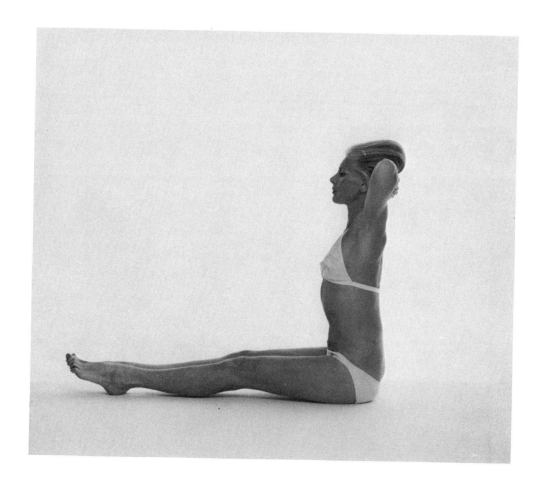

more momentum, then, once you have come up, reach over and touch your toes, but that is for beginners. As soon as possible, make this a gut issue and force your hip flexor and abdominal muscles to take the full load.

If you cannot keep your legs on the floor as you sit up, anchor your ankles or calves under a stable piece of furniture or have someone hold them down.

Inhale as you come up, exhale at peak, and continue to exhale as you uncurl and bring every inch of your abdominals into play, firming the lower as well as the upper range.

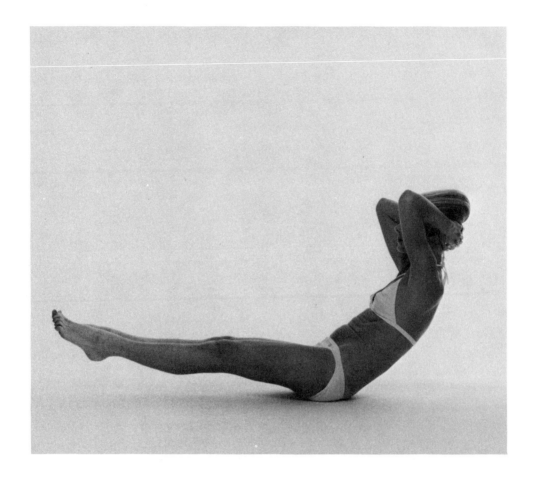

The most important part of this exercise is not sitting up but how you ease back to the floor. It is this second phase that really forces the abdominals to harden in order to sustain your slow-motion descent. If you collapse like a rag doll, your belly will derive little benefit.

Instead, the trick is to tense and hold at least twice on your way down. I do so at roughly 10 and 20 minutes past the hour, calculating sitting position as high noon. When you are in champion form, you can also hold at 12:28 without your abdominals getting the shakes.

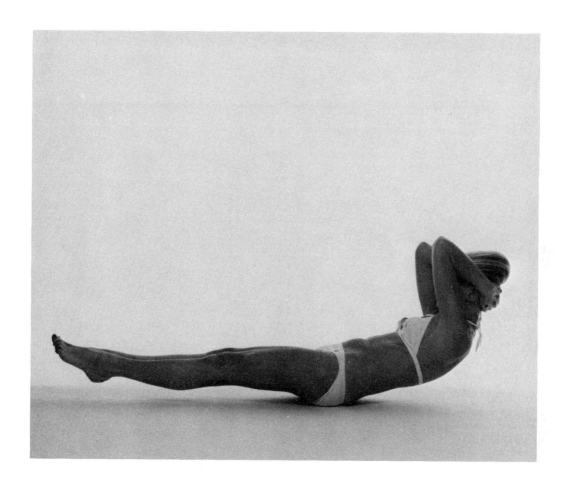

Normally one is taught to complete the cycle with legs and feet never leaving the floor. I sometimes do it that way. For variety, and because I find it gives an extra pull, I lift my legs at the first hold and lower them gradually.

This system gives an extra pull because it obliges you to maintain balance as well—your abdominals have to cope with both ends at once. If that is too much and you lose control, keep your legs on the floor. Start sit-ups at whatever count your body can take, eventually building up to 50.

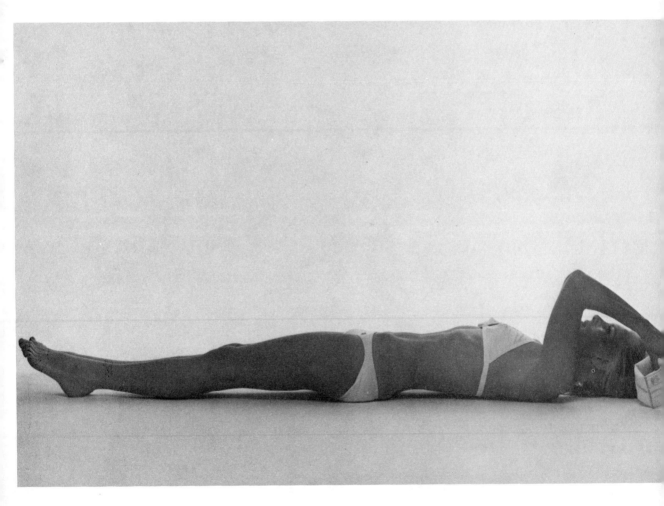

78

The Applause Muscle

Time for a rest. Let your lower body sink blissfully into the mat —it has done enough for the day. All you have to worry about now is one reluctant, deprived muscle that you never think twice about until suddenly it begins to flap in the breeze. Good-bye, sleeveless dresses! I wish beauty did not demand such unflagging attention to detail, but it does.

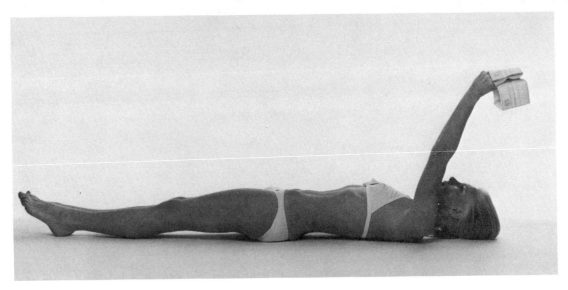

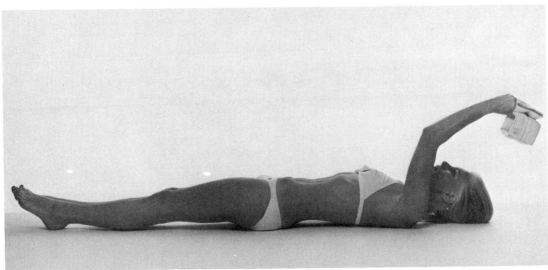

80

Flexible weight or weights in hand, you take care of the inner part of your upper arms by using it like a pump. Lift the weight by extending your arm. Slowly lower. Repeat 20 times at the minimum. Switch to your other arm. To make it tougher—and get it over more quickly —do both arms at once.

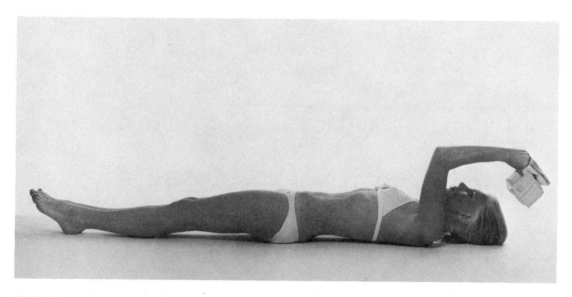

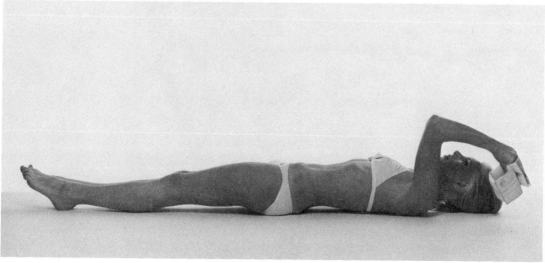

The Side Stretch

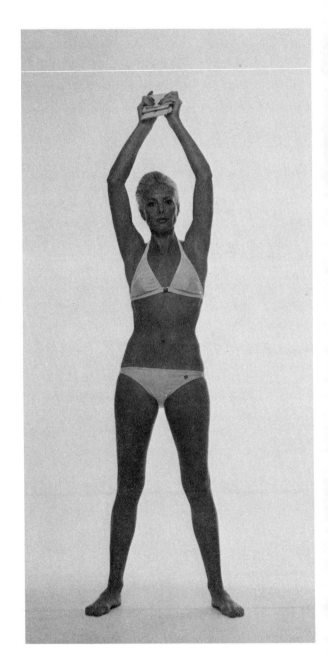

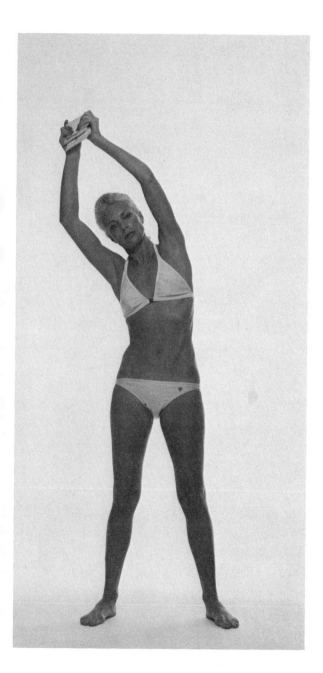

By now you are ready to stand on your own two feet and pull out the kinks. The side stretch trims the waistline while firming the arms. (Should your legs still feel tense from the workout they have been through, as you first stand up, lift one leg and give it a shake, then the other.)

The custom is to start an exercise series with a stretch so that you warm up before proceeding to tougher, more specific movements. So if you wish, go ahead and start with this rather than with your thigh routine. Personally, I prefer to begin lying down and warm up as I go along. Once my thighs are done, the rest is a lark.

To do the side stretch, preferably with weights, reach for the sky with both hands as high as you can go. Feel your rib cage lift, tuck in your bottom, and pull in your stomach. Even if you are short and squat, you suddenly grow skinny and tall; if you are a beanpole, you are no longer one that droops.

I show the successive stages of the stretch, though in this case there is no need to hold. The exercise should be done in a rapid, uninterrupted arc. The photographs show the correct position. You must bend to the side, not lean forward. That way you feel the pull down to the hip.

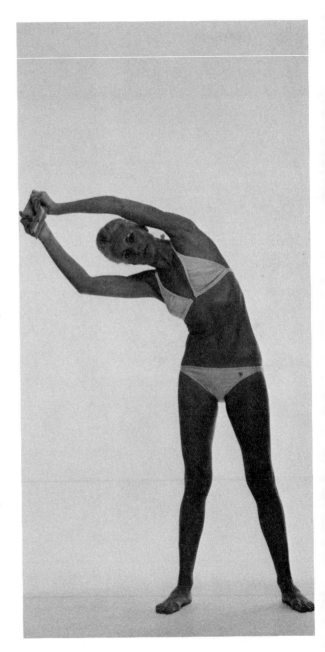

84

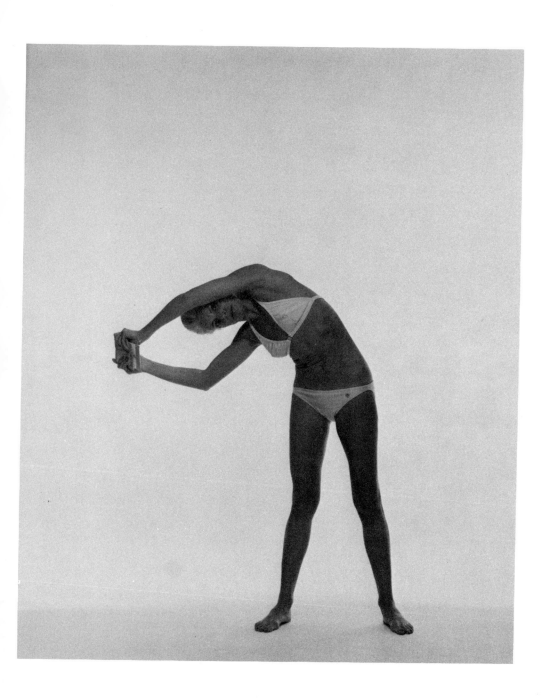

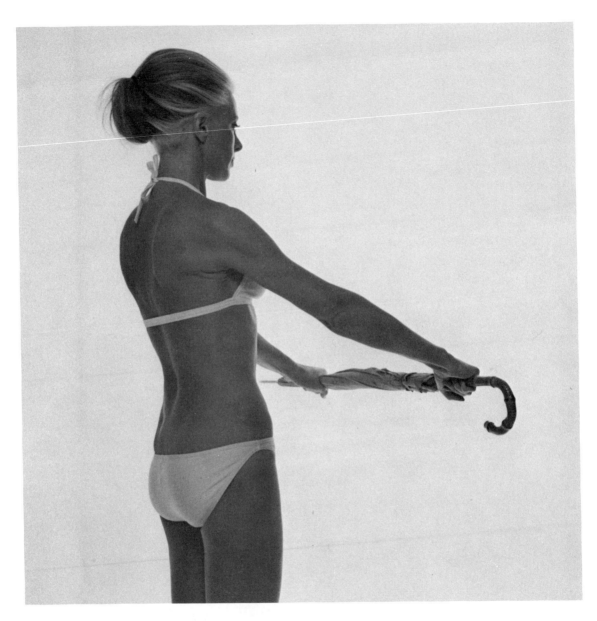

The Pectoral Squeeze

Don't take a raincheck on your bosom—grab that umbrella now. To flesh out a bony chest or keep up your Mae West specials, good pectorals are indispensable. Forget that mail-order gear and put your muscles to work. You won't gain inches, or recover lost buoyancy—like a soufflé, once your breasts fall they don't rise again—but you may lose your hang-up about wearing décolletage; you will look so much better in a low neckline.

Firm pectorals are the only gay deceivers because they are for real, and if you have small breasts they are the only bra you need. Large breasts require both good muscle tone and a good bra.

At some point we all fail the pencil test—when the pencil placed at the under curve of the breast no longer falls. So what! Would you rather have prostate problems?

To firm your pectoral muscles, take an old umbrella (or a broomstick or a plant dowel) and, with arms extended roughly at hip level, squeeze it as though you were wringing it out. This gives you a contraction on both sides from inner elbow through to the breastbone. Relax and lift the umbrella above your head, squeeze, and relax—the contraction affects your side muscles (they, too, are supportive unless allowed to become lazy).

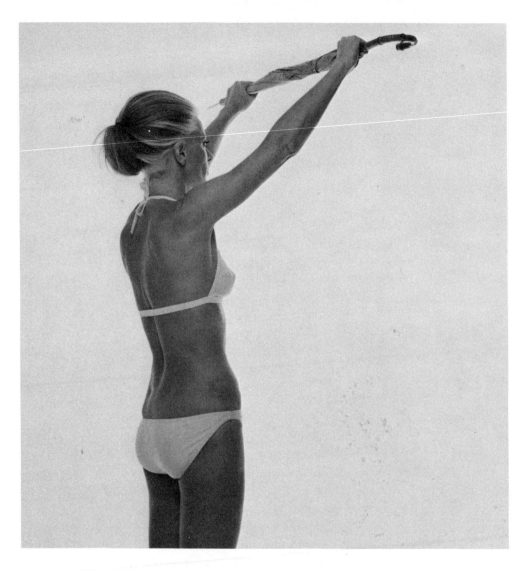

Lower the umbrella to shoulder
height. Squeeze, and the frontal
muscles tense again, giving your
breasts an automatic lift and
thrust forward. Repeat the cycle
20 times or more, depending on
need. Once you have located the
muscles involved, through
specific exercise, it will become a
habit to contract and relax them
at random moments during the
day. You sense you are slumping,
feel your nipples are headed
south, and without raising your
shoulders you bring up your breasts
(and your head) by contracting
your pectorals. Your back also
straightens up, and you feel better.

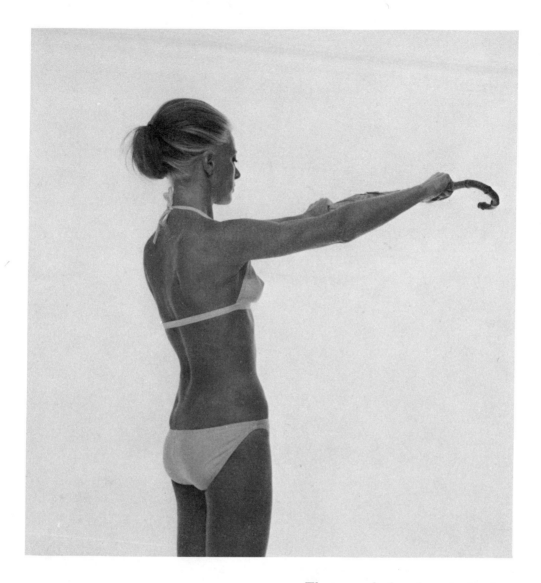

That concludes the mimimal
beauty workout. For alternatives
and reinforcements, see the
following exercises, listed by
category.

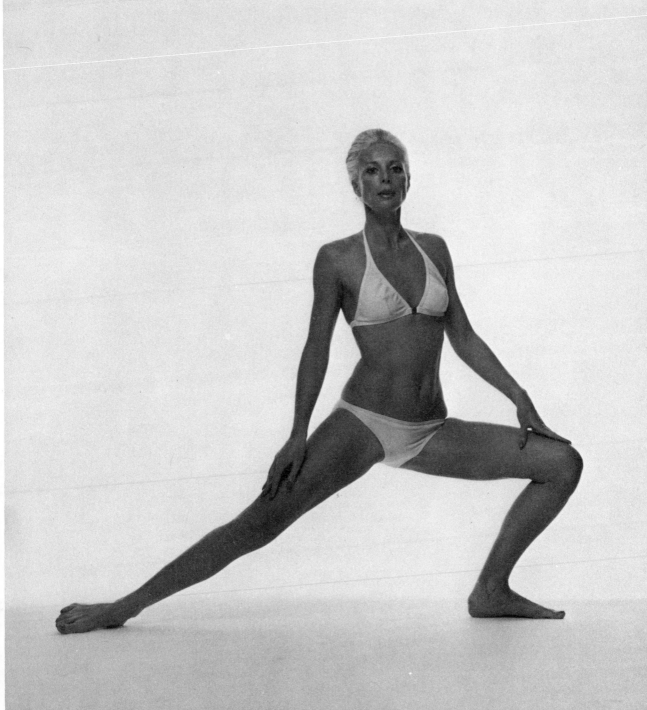

Jaunty Bottom, Beautiful Thighs

What is the most common figure complaint? "If I put on two pounds, it sinks straight to my rear end." Sister, I am with you—the problem seems to be built in unless you are built like a man. I have been exercising regularly now for over fifteen years in order to avoid a pear shape, but the potential is always there. A little neglect leads straight to a lot of behind.

The next most common affliction is cellulite. Even without swings in weight, women are prone to this unattractive form of fat. I don't ask for thighs of bronze—who wants to grab those—but nonetheless it is maddening when they deteriorate. You figure you must be doing something right because the rest of you looks fine—so why are you suddenly afflicted with jelly on the thigh?

To recognize where you are vulnerable is the first line of defense.

The number of my exercises devoted to well-rounded thighs and buttocks is large, precisely because that is where your body, left untended, thickens and wobbles.

The Fanny Lift

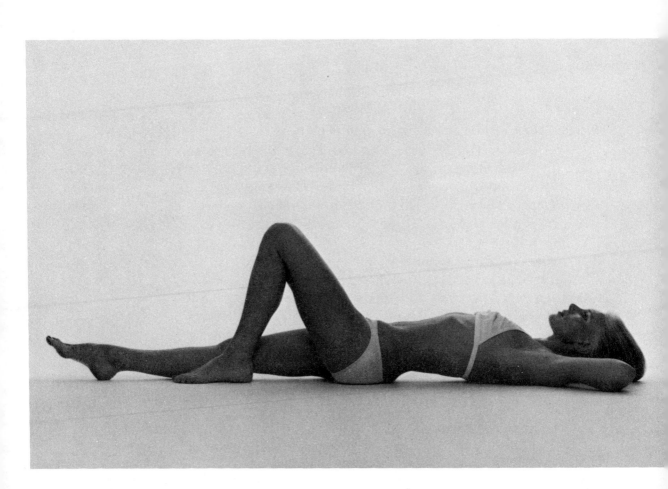

Designed for your backside, this exercise also firms the thighs. Sometimes I wear ankle weights, sometimes I don't, to remind myself to be less concerned with my legs and think Annie Fanny here. The two are connected, but the emphasis shifts. Lie down,

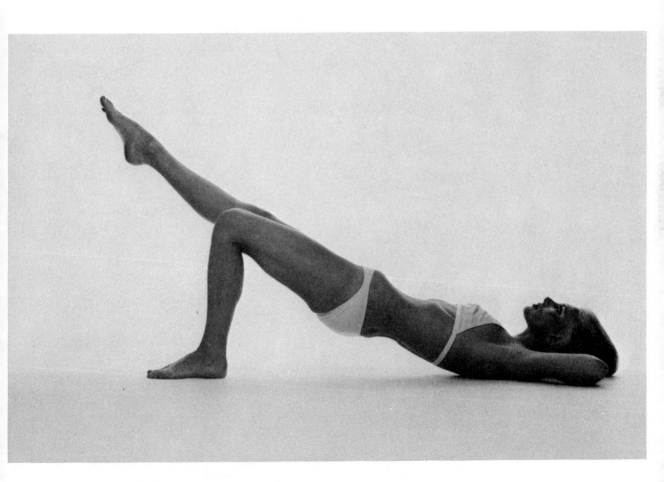

arms behind your head, one leg bent at the knee. Take a deep breath, exhale. Inhale normally, kick with the other leg, and lift the body off the floor. The foot of the bent leg and your shoulders and head keep you on keel. Very important: at the top of the kick exhale, tighten your buttocks, and hold. Pretend you have just done a heist and that is where you've stashed the loot.

Don't be deceived by appearances. As in most exercises involving the upper leg and behind, the initial thrust

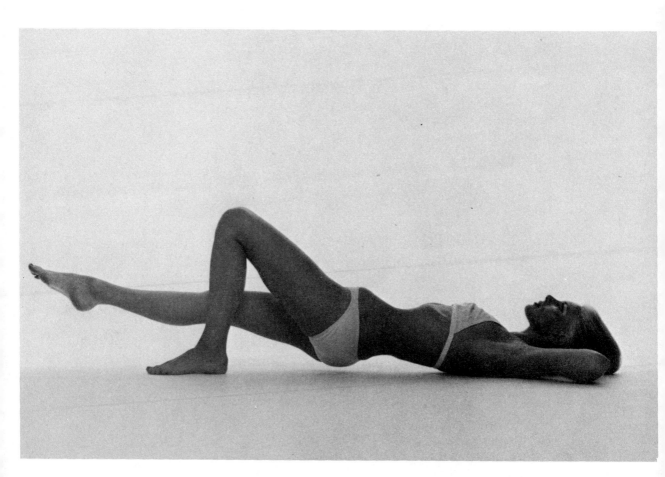

looks like the major effort. Instead, it is the easiest part. We are dealing with major, supportive muscles, and the only way to keep them strong is to put them under stress. For example, anyone in decent condition can lunge forward like a fencer. But can you sustain the position without the thrust muscle trembling like a leaf?

In the fanny lift, you lower slowly, buttocks still tight. You will feel it in the bent leg as well as the extended leg. Repeat 20 to 50 times, then reverse legs.

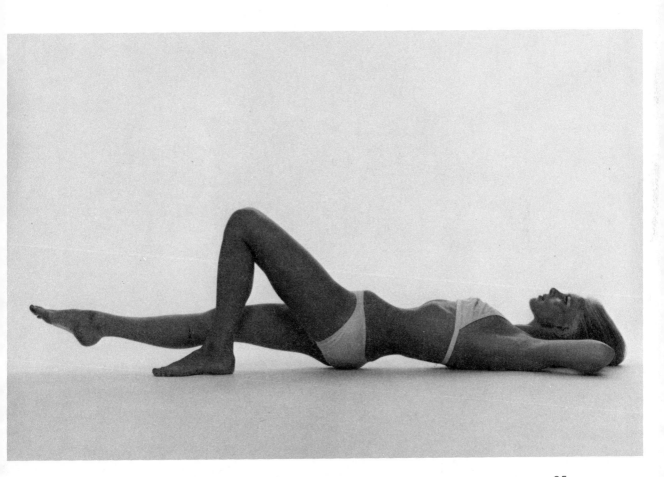

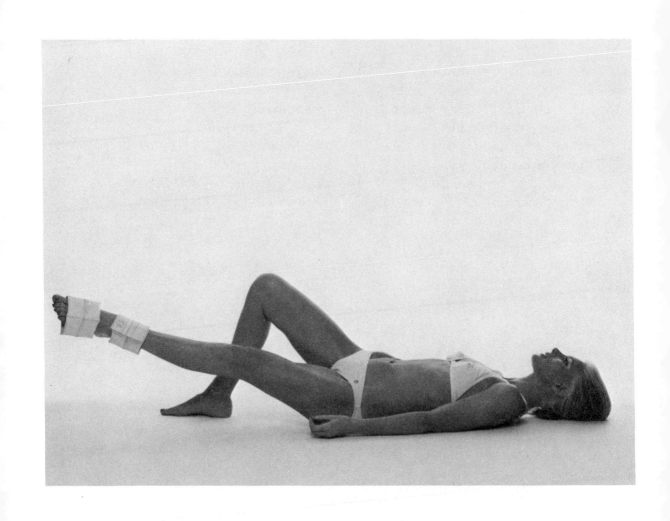

The Leg Lift

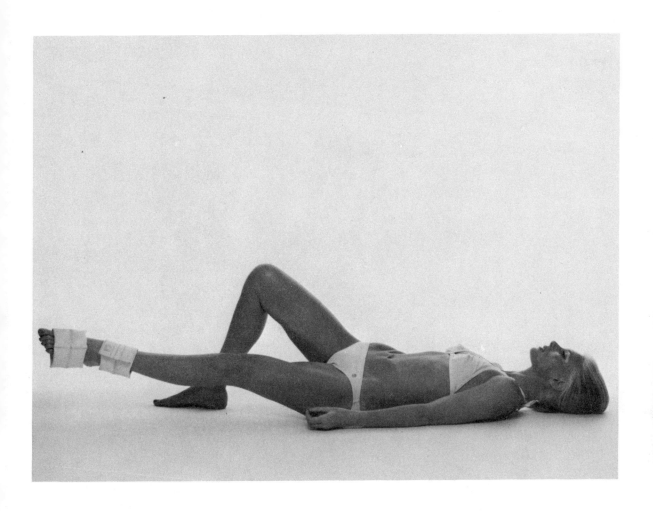

I wear weights to make my legs—and abdomen—work harder. The lift-and-lower motion is similar to the preceding fanny lift, and, to vary your program, I suggest you do these exercises on alternate days. I am sure you have seen pictures of both legs being raised simultaneously, as well as the gym variation where you suspend

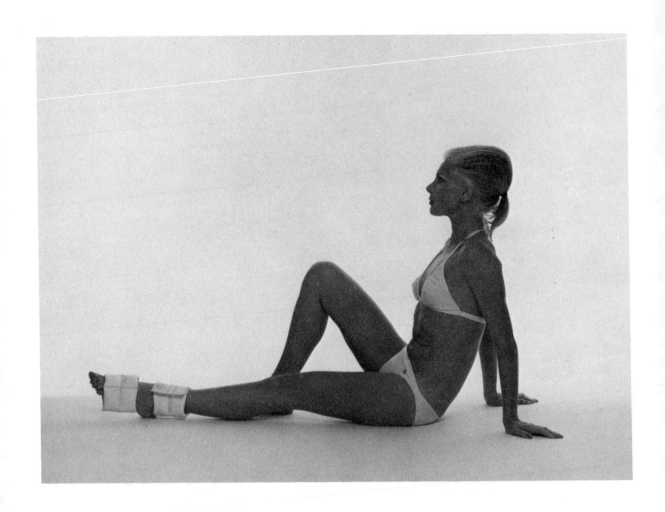

yourself by grabbing a bar and
hoist both dangling legs to waist
level. If you are in good enough
shape for either, skip the leg lift.
You're too athletic to need it. The
trouble with lifting both legs off
the floor together, which is

sometimes prescribed as a
post-pregnancy exercise, is that
without strong abdominals you
may strain the middle back. After
childbirth your abdominals have
to be toned. They can't do their
job, so your back arches off the

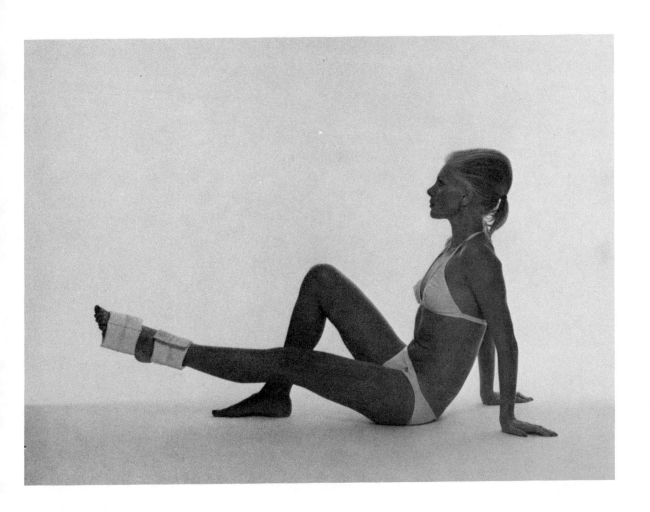

floor and you weaken it, thereby compounding your problem: your abdomen stays flabby and your back goes out of line as well.

Should you feel back strain, even in my mild approach, put a small pillow under your hips.

That is in the easy lie-back position. The same lift done sitting up gives more of a pull on the lower abdomen. It is up to you to judge how much you can take. Your thighs will benefit either way.

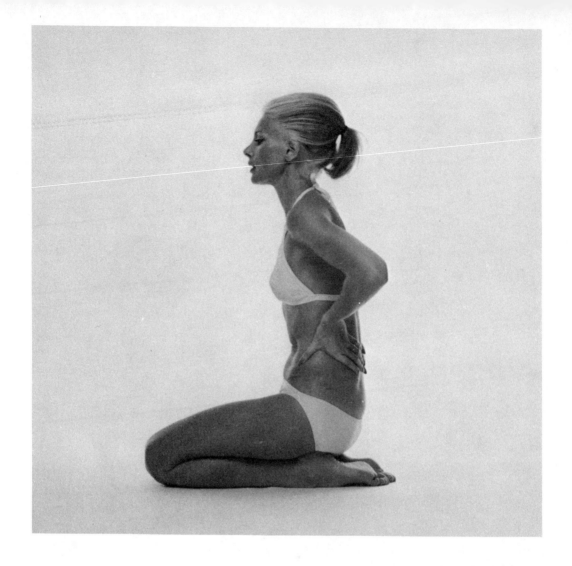

Frontal
Assault

Sit with your legs tucked under
you, bottom resting easily and
abdomen flat. All you have to do
is raise yourself off the floor. It
looks very simple and is, except
for one catch. Your hands are
placed just above the hips to

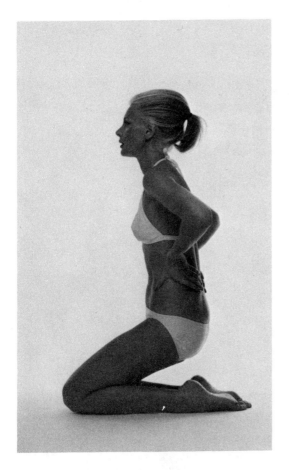
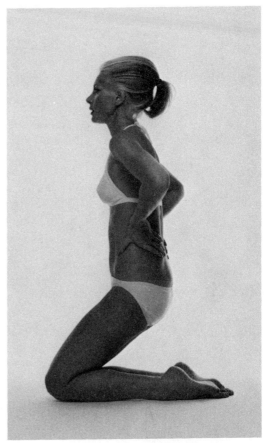

repress the instinct to lead with your behind. No protruding fanny here (or slanted back, or head tilted forward); that accomplishes nothing.

You want to come up straight. I call the exercise Frontal Assault because the propulsion comes from the front of the thighs. To condition the muscle, you come up slowly and return by degrees.

Don't sit each time. Keep moving. If the muscle shrieks, let it; it is the sort that can take it, but do not prolong the stress in the beginning. Start with 10 to 20 times and increase number and degree of slowness gradually. You may not obtain the supple force of a dancer's frontal thigh, but this is a classic warm-up exercise for modern dance.

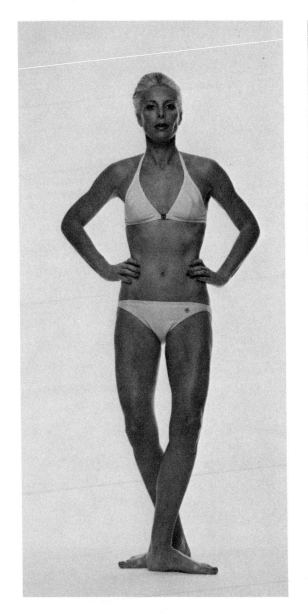
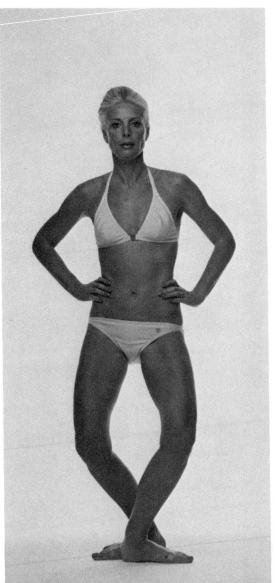

102

The Pliers

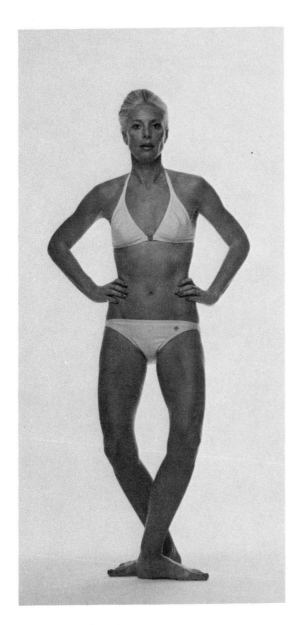

Forgive the pun. The Pliers also derives from dance, in this case the demi-plié, except that I place my feet in third ballet position rather than first. It is easier and just as effective for tightening the thighs.

Once mastered this way, it can be done in first position: feet heel to heel with toes pointing east and west from the body; or in fifth: heel to toes. Each position gives a slight shift in balance and tension.

I place my hands on my hips again to monitor my alignment: pelvis tilted forward, bottom in, and abdomen flat.

You have guessed it. The exercise is done in smooth, continuous slow motion—no jerking up and down. At first you may creak, but the aim is effortless grace. After a count of 20 (or more), reverse legs and repeat.

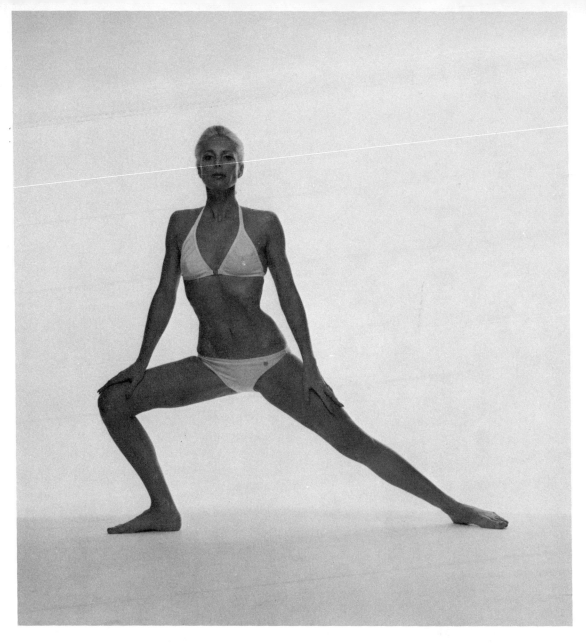

The Lunge

Stand with legs wide apart, thighs turned out if possible. The point is to feel at ease and ready to lunge with poise from one side to the other, 20 to 40 times. Those

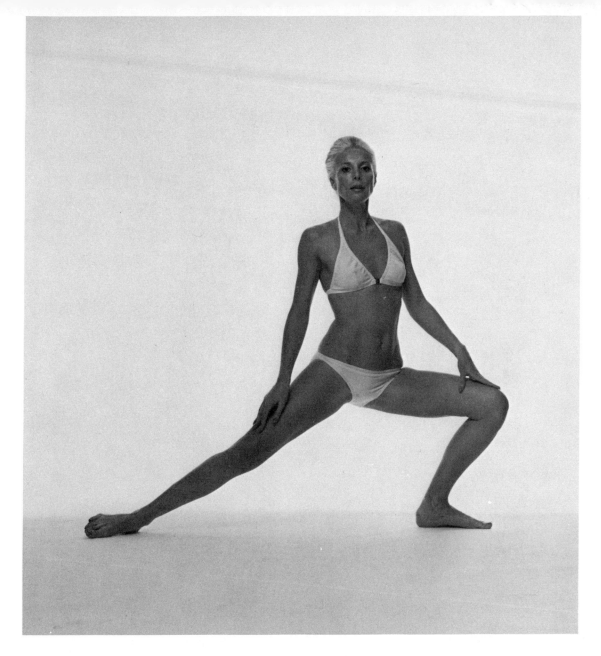

with arthritic knees should abstain, and don't push weak knees so far that they hurt. Assuming you have no such problems, this exercise may prevent them, and it's fantastic for your inner thighs.

I think it is fun. You get carried away by your own momentum, and the lower you go, the better—as long as you are in control. Don't go so far that you cannot pull back up without breaking the rhythm.

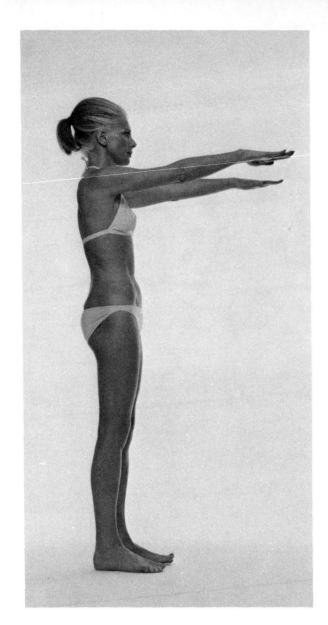
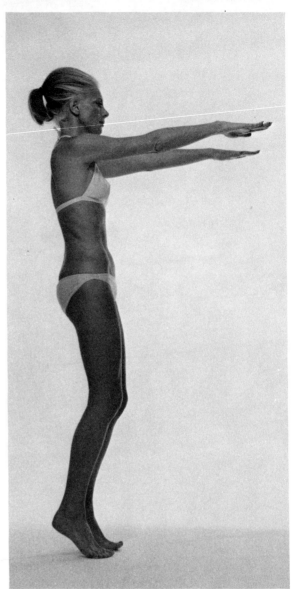

Deep Knee
Bends

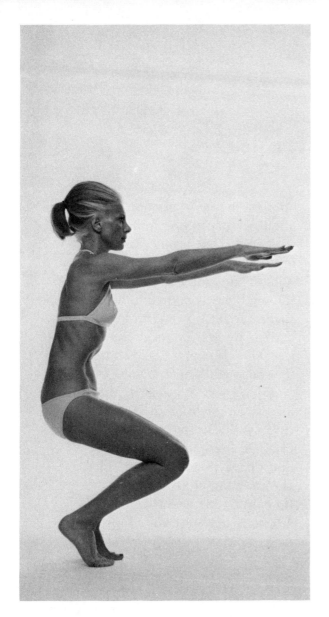

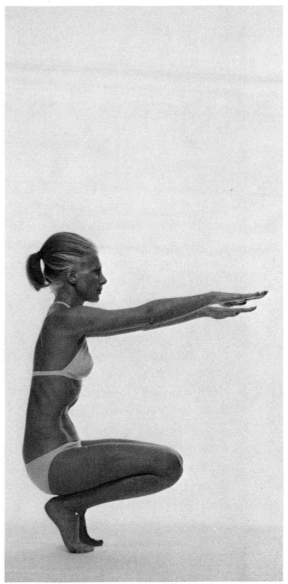

This old chestnut remains a favorite of mine because it improves balance as well as thighs. To help keep my balance, I focus on a fixed object across the room.

Arms should be raised parallel at shoulder height and the back kept straight. Arching the back throws you off balance. Don't worry about creaking as you go up and down, though again, if your knees really ache, stop; 20 is plenty.

The Hammer

This is a variation of the Back Stroke shown in the minimal beauty workout and serves as an alternate. It is equally good for tightening the backside and the back of the thighs; and it also firms the long frontal-thigh muscle.

Sometimes I point the lifted toe, sometimes I hold it parallel to the floor. *Plus ça change, plus c'est la même chose*, yet every little difference reawakens alertness to muscle. As you become accustomed to an exercise, you tend to run through it mechanically. The trick is to keep the exercise fresh and challenging, so that you think about what you are doing.

Stretch out prone, head cradled in your arms, hammer leg bent at the knee. Inhale. Raise the leg high. Exhale and hold. Bring the leg down with force, but hold again just before touching the floor. Imagine that you have a stubborn nail and a fragile "wall" you don't want to mar, or that you are accomplishing an esoteric rite: symbolically you have crushed the opposition, so you don't have to do it in fact. The Hammer should barely graze the floor, then lift again. Do it 20 to 40 times, and alternate legs.

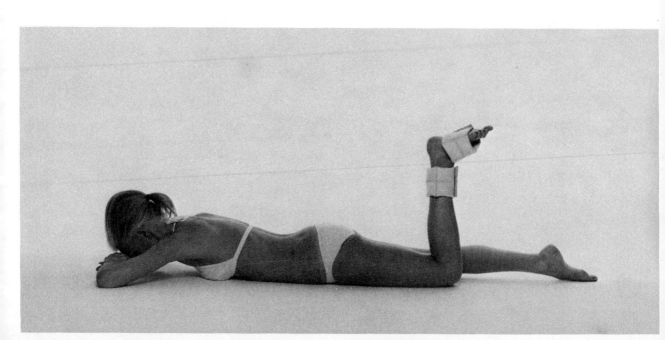

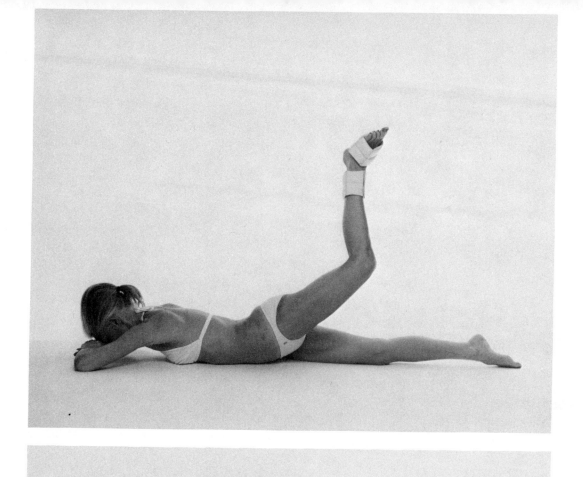

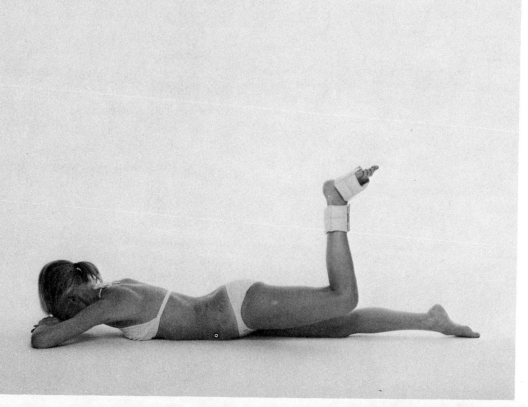

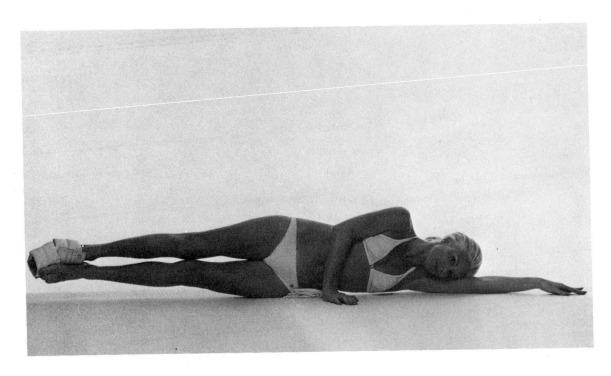

Double Trouble

Are you bored with the simple Side Kick? Try Double Trouble. Along with combating saddlebags on your outer thighs, this lift narrows your waist. You should feel the pull all the way up to your ribs. (The inner thigh will also tense with the effort.)

You need one bent arm with hand on the floor for support here. Otherwise you will find that your legs are swinging forward or backward: they should be raised together, toes touching, straight up to the side. Inhale as you lift, exhale as you lower, sustaining the descent. Do this 20 to 40 times. Roll over and repeat.

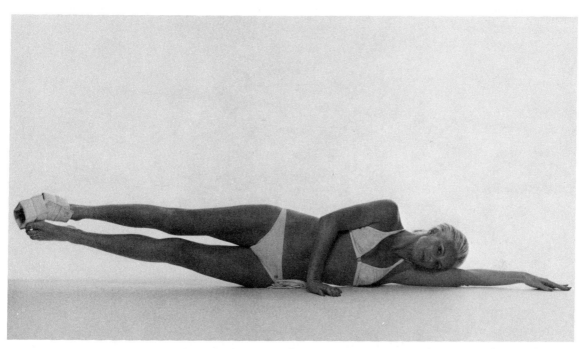

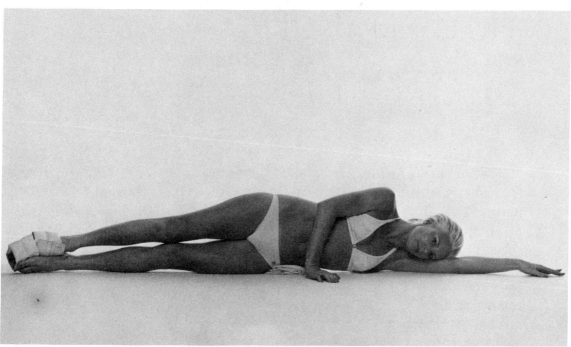

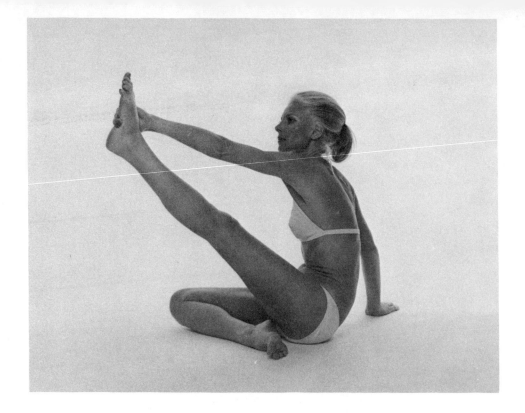

The Thigh
Stretch

No weights here. The aim is
elongation and suppleness,
particularly of the inner thigh. It
is a perfect way to conclude a
series of leg exercises: your
muscles are warmed up, they
have worked hard, and now you
are giving them a parting elegant
stretch. At first it may seem more
like a wrench, but never mind.

Sit on the floor with your right
leg bent so that the foot curls
under the opposite thigh, placing
your right arm to the back of you
for support. Bend your left leg,
grab your left foot by the arch
with your left hand, and raise and
extend the leg to the fullest, as
wide and as high as you can go.
Do not let your right knee jerk off

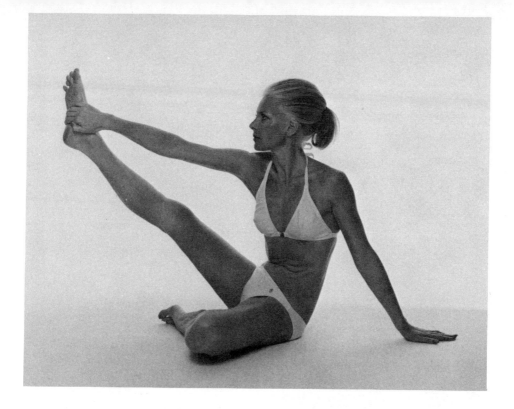

the floor; if anything, press the right knee against the floor to give the other leg more expansion. Reverse position, extend your right leg. Continue left, right, left, right, 20 times. Do more, if you wish, but 20, even 10, are enough to stretch the muscle.

Depending on the state of your knees, the exercise can be varied by folding the leg that is not being extended tailor-fashion to the back of you. This stretches that thigh as well, but do not do it if you feel strain on the knee. Not that knees should not be exercised—as with any joints, bending and straightening are part of their function; nonetheless, if knees creak from lack of exercise, take it easy. This applies even to the extended leg. It should go up and out straight, without locking the knee. Don't use force; if not at once, little by little you will get there. We are all in different condition. I used to find this exercise difficult and was determined to make it a habit. To my astonishment, lots of people find it a snap. Maybe they did the French can-can in their youth, and compared to that, it is a cinch. Remember the French can-can step where, while keeping your balance on one foot, you grab the other by the arch, pull that leg up to your ear, and twirl, ruffles flying and garter displayed?

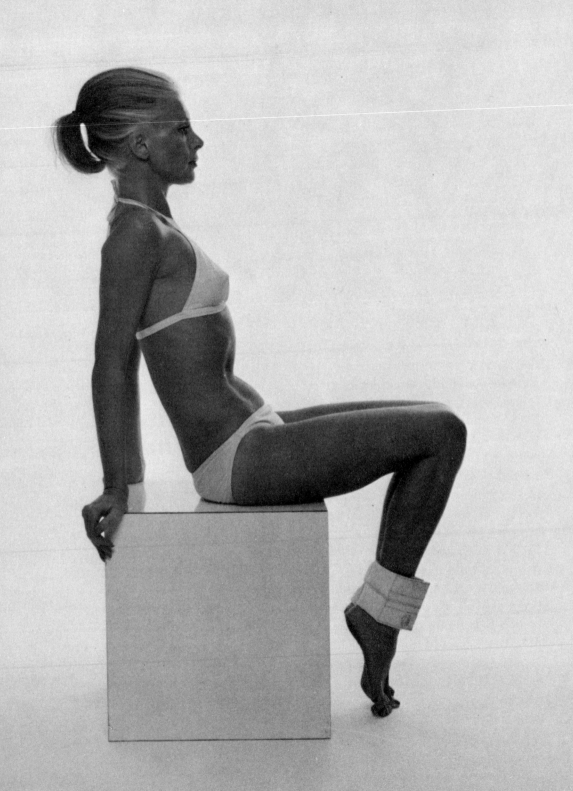

Abominable Abdominals

It is foolish not to keep your abdominal muscles in shape. Gluttony, pregnancy, desk work, or laziness are not excuses. Heavy thighs are not necessarily unhealthy, but a paunch is bad for you, as well as being unattractive. So is slackening, which is hard to discern when you are covered up, but visible in the nude, as well you know. In fact, in the latter case—the model's syndrome—you may begin to have weird stomachaches and cramps, often diagnosed as psychosomatic, when the true culprit is bad muscle tone. For lack of proper support, your insides drop and complain.

Succumbing to middle-aged spread, you may start to flounder in bloat and become the sort of jolly figure your dear ones can live with but only a mother could love.

For a landslide stomach, include at least two abdominal exercises in your exercise program: the sit-ups in the minimal beauty workout, plus one of the following. Try all of these in turn to keep your muscles alert. Once through the repertoire, start from the beginning again. What you thought you had mastered presents fresh difficulty when it's no longer familiar.

Meanwhile, as your muscle control and awareness increase, form the habit of tensing and pulling in your middle while walking, standing, and so on. The better your basic posture, the less you have to correct through special exercise.

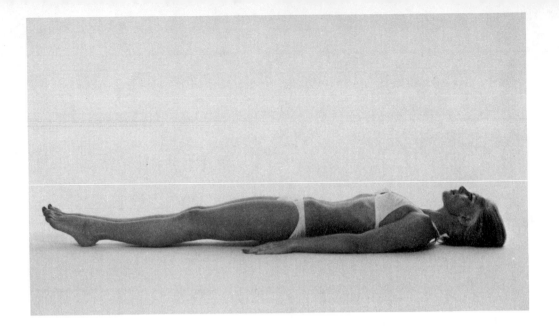

The Ankle Grab

I always like to do this one. It gives a sense of equilibrium that is more than physical because it implies body balance. To stay on keel, you have to know how to rock on your lower spine. That is not your usual perch except when you slump on a sofa. No slumping, no sofa here.

Arms at your sides, flat on your back, inhale and begin by raising both torso and legs. Feel the pull on your abdominals. Push on, bending your knees and extending your arms so your hands briefly grab your ankles in the air. Hold, more or less poised on your coccyx (the small bone at the base of the spinal column). Exhale.

Do not fall back in a heap on the floor. Gradually, lower torso and legs, gripping your outer thighs if need be to steady yourself. Again, feel the pull in the belly. Flatten out on the floor. Repeat 10, 20, 50 times.

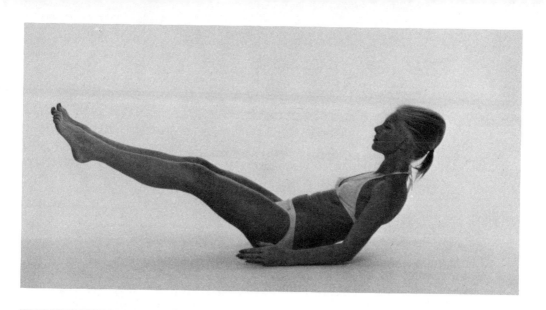

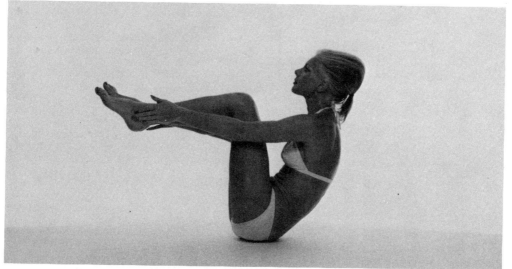

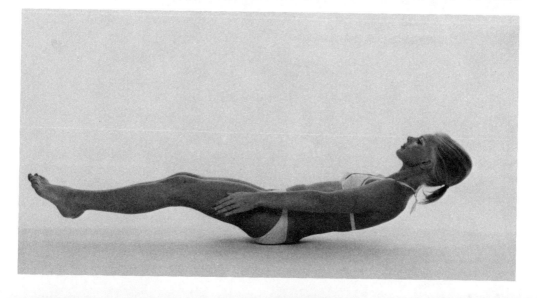

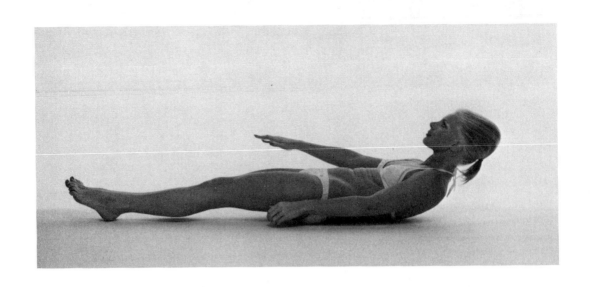

Tip to Toe

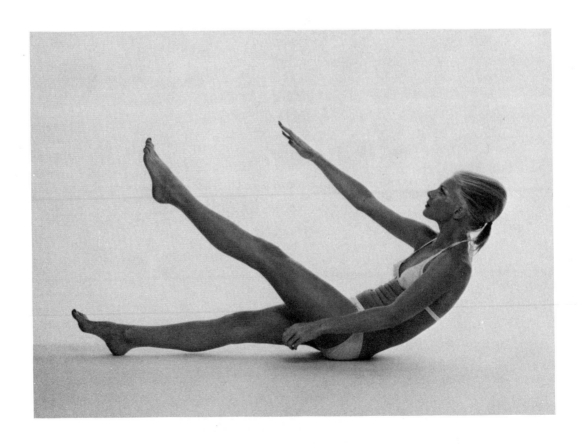

Raising one leg at a time is not as tough on the abdominals as raising both simultaneously. However, it puts them to work, and the high kick helps firm the thigh.

From supine position, lift right arm and upper torso. Continue to lift and swing up your left leg so that fingertips and toes touch briefly. Both the swung and the reclining leg should be straight, with the latter clinging to the floor.

Exhale at touch point, then unfold to supine position, slowly for maximum benefit. After 20 to 40 times, alternate leg and arm and repeat.

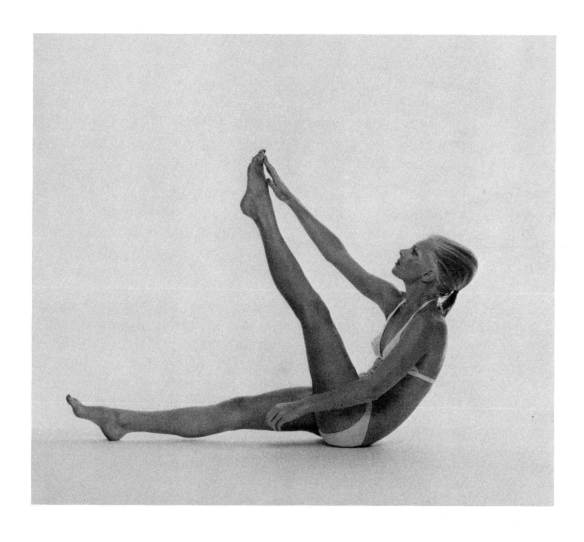

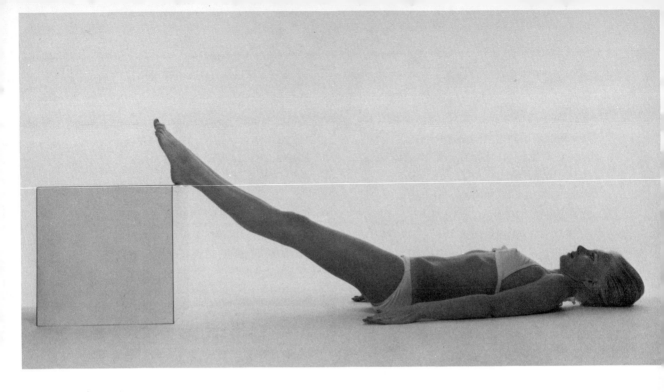

The Jackknife

Whether or not it looks it, this exercise is easier than ordinary sit-ups that require keeping your legs, including your knees, straight out on the floor. As you know, if you cannot keep your legs down, you train yourself by having someone sit on them or by placing the ankles under a heavy piece of furniture.

Before your ankles turn black and blue, try this alternative. Once you have mastered it, you can go back to sit-ups. I do the Jackknife on days that I am tired,

or when I have concentrated on other hip and abdominal workouts. All exercises that involve lifting the torso off the floor give the hips a real workout.

Legs propped up on a cube or kitchen chair, arms at your sides, inhale, raise arms and torso swiftly. Touch pointed toes with extended fingers. Return, prolonging the agony as much as possible by halting as you go. Repeat until abdominals quiver. With practice, you build endurance.

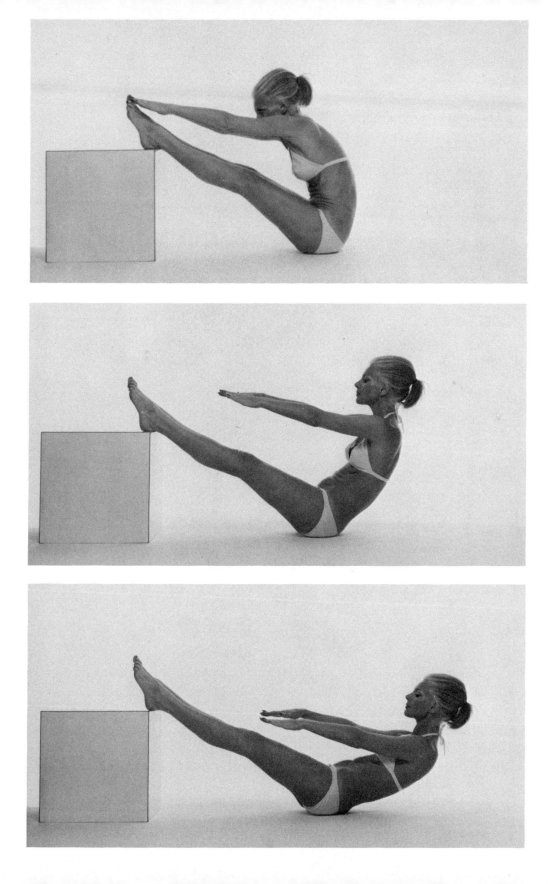

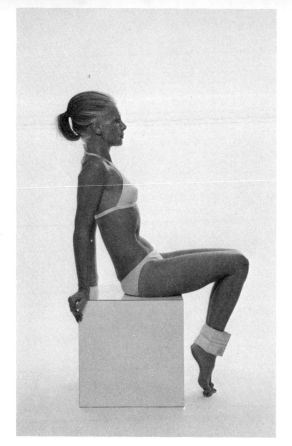
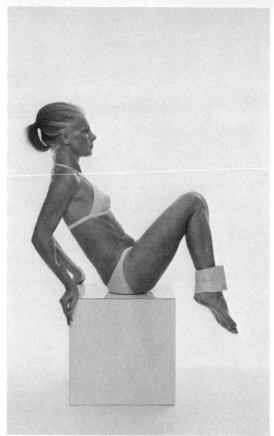

Legs Up,
Mother Brown

Theoretically, you can do this in a dull moment at the office, though office exercise usually never pans out—and I don't recommend it on a swivel chair. Executed properly, Legs Up strengthens the outer side of your abdominal muscles as well as all the area in between.

Grip the back of a sturdy chair for balance and support, suspending legs in the air. Very slowly twist to the right, twist to

122

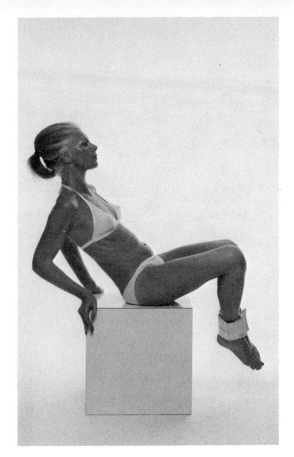

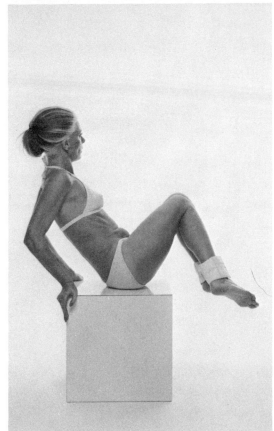

the left, return to center, and lower legs until toes touch the floor. Hold just before touching in a final hurrah.

You may be able to twist better and with more composure than I display here. While twisting, you may hear your lower vertebrae crack. That is a good sign—they need it to keep the spine supple, and an easy crackle and pop saves a sudden awful snap.

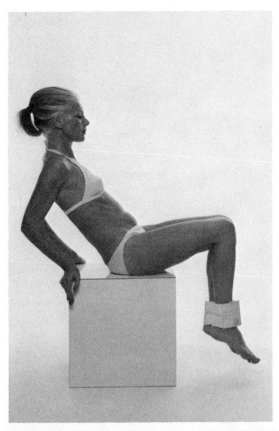

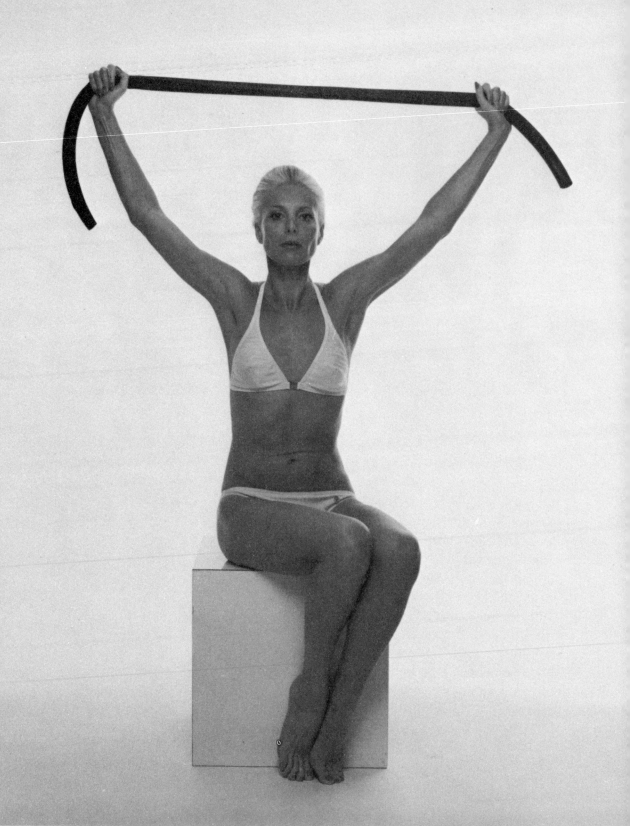

Pectoral Perks

An old inner tube is your bosom's best friend. The tube gets stretched and you stay firm. Even with breasts beyond recall —or not worth mentioning, like mine—good pectoral tone gives a look of buoyancy. That is the look you want to maintain: roundness as opposed to flatness or sag.

Forget about your breasts and build your pectorals. There is no sense padding yourself with a bra if your upper chest has caved in. The contrast is obvious. On the other hand, with good shoulders and a smoothly muscled upper chest the lift works, and meantime you have created true built-in support.

Proper carriage and breathing are also the secret of breast maintenance, no matter what the size. Regular exercise, including the trick of consciously tightening and relaxing the pectorals during the day, does the rest.

Boob Tube Ahoy!

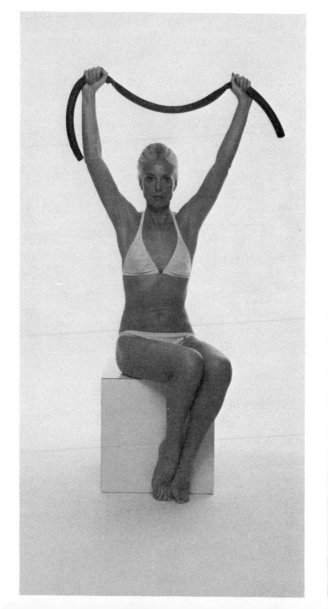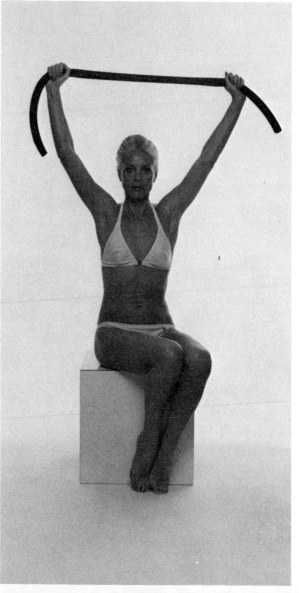

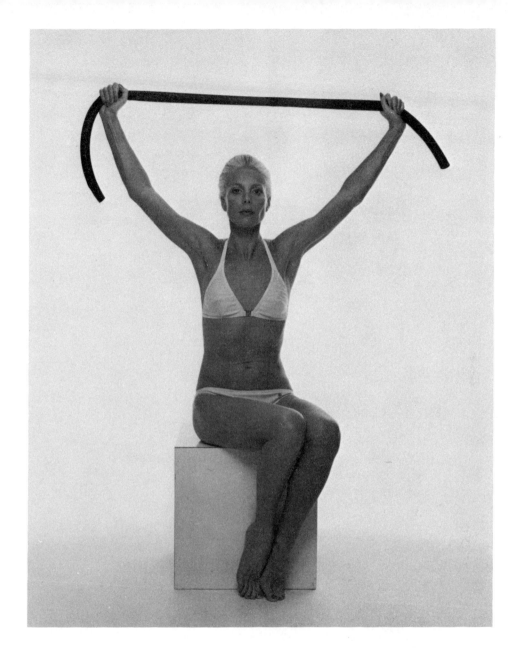

Raise the tube high, though limp, grasping it firmly. Inhale and pull it taut, then stretch it to maximum. Excellent for breasts, shoulders, forearms, and upper back. Exhale and repeat 20 to 40 times. While at maximum, I also suggest you do a quick abdominal contraction. It comes naturally and extends the scope of the exercise, firming two areas at once.

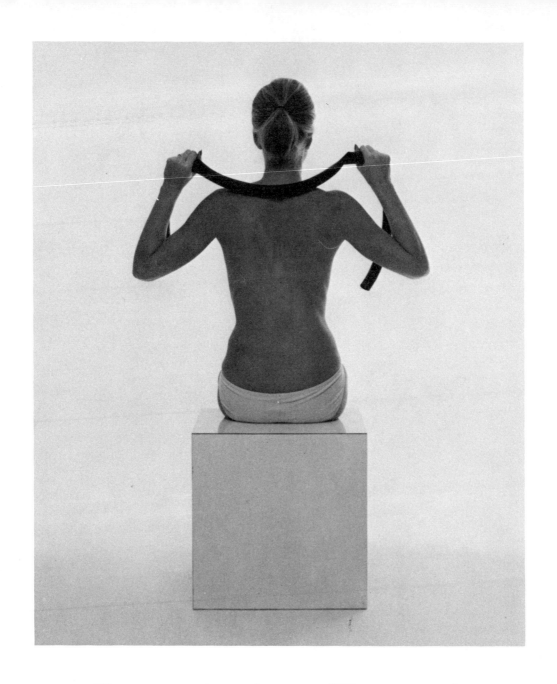

Back to Front

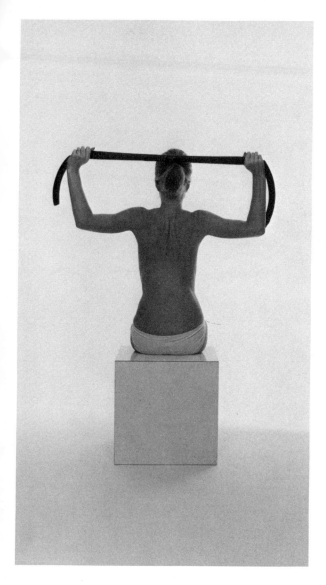
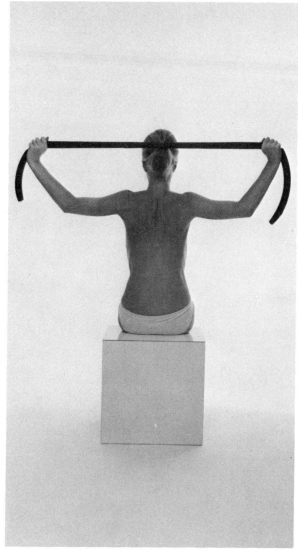

Loop the inner tube around the
back of your neck as if you were
putting on a boa. Get a good grip
on it. Lift to mid-head, meanwhile
stretching the tube so that it
forms a rectangle with your bent
arms held at shoulder height.
Give another yank on the tube,
pulling it out as far as you can.
Not only do your pectorals harden
and your breasts stick up and out,
you should feel the tension in
your forearms, shoulders, and
upper back: all of which
contribute to a pretty décolletage.
Do it 20 to 40 times.

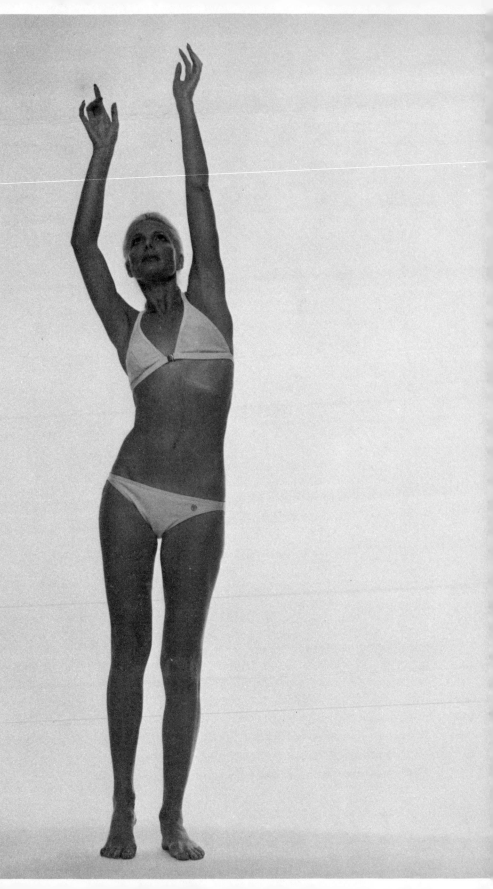

Home Stretch

The aim of beauty exercises is not to be muscle-bound and rigid. Your goal is strong but elongated muscle that gives you support and a smooth contour. You don't want to bulge; in fact, you might be dismayed if someone were to compliment you on your muscle—and not on your terrific figure.

Yes, you will have muscle after all the exercise you have done. But you will also have a sleeker, more flexible body.

For sleekness and flexibility, stretches are perhaps even more important than the heavy work, although the two complement each other. You build with weights, then achieve lightness by bending and pulling, like taffy. Working with weights is a necessary chore; stretches are a pleasure.

Stretches also vary; some are designed to trim the body, others help you relax. I have included both kinds.

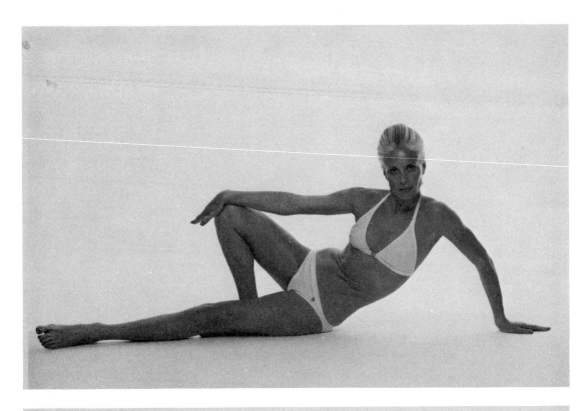

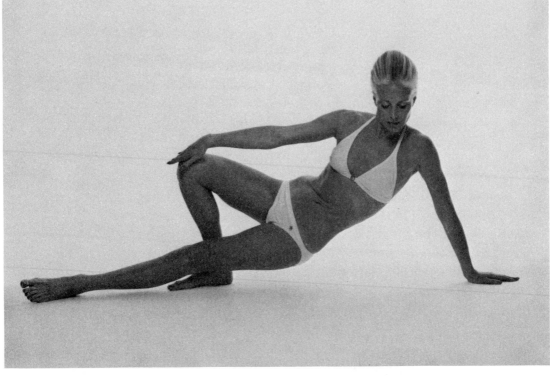

The Side Pull

As you lift up, you should feel the pull all the way to the armpit as your whole side gets a good stretch; meanwhile you are strengthening the muscles of your supporting leg and arm.

The leg of the side to be lifted should be straight on the floor and straight when raised—without full extension, the exercise is less effective. As you assume initial position, don't let the leg loll. On the contrary, try to inch the foot just beyond where you would normally place it for comfort.

You raise, lower in continuous, moderately rapid succession, holding an instant at summit. Do this 20 to 40 times, change sides, and repeat.

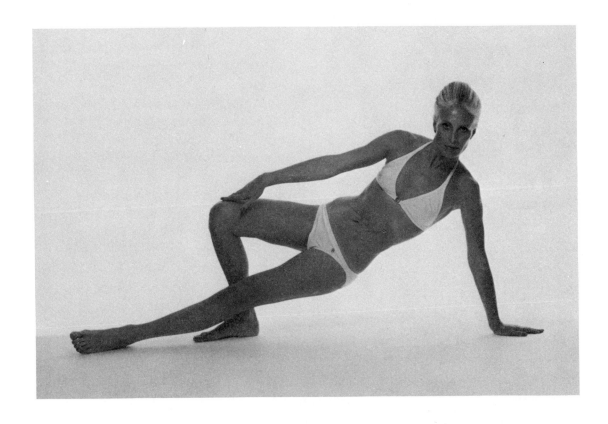

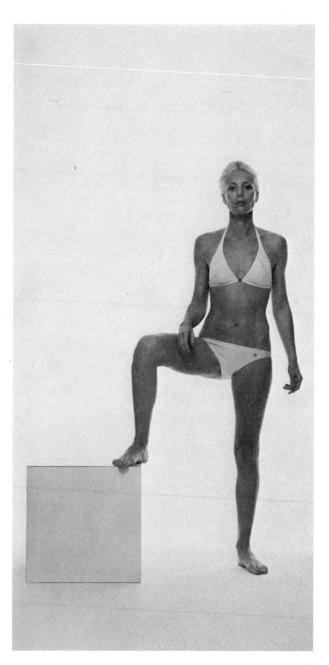

Touch the Floor

I prefer this to the usual straight-forward bend and touch your toes. The split-level approach gives more of a stretch to the leg on the floor, as well as a scrunch to the thigh of the hoisted leg. For the cube shown here you can substitute the rung or the seat of a chair.

I suppose for an extra pull I could raise my arms above my head before reaching down to the ground. I don't because starting with arms loose at standing position reminds me each time I reach point zero to tuck in my hips and put my body in line.

Up, down, up, down—smooth and easy does it. When it becomes too simple to touch only in front of your foot, reach and touch by your heel. Do it 20 times, change legs, and dip again.

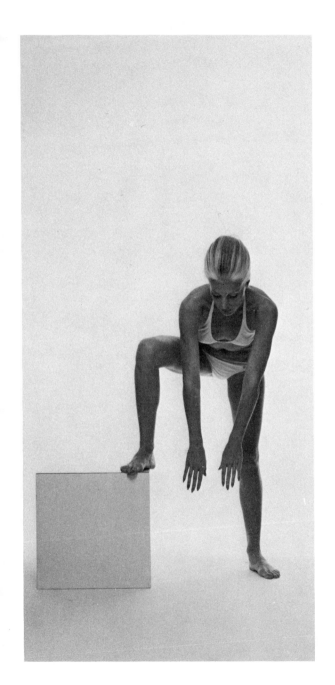
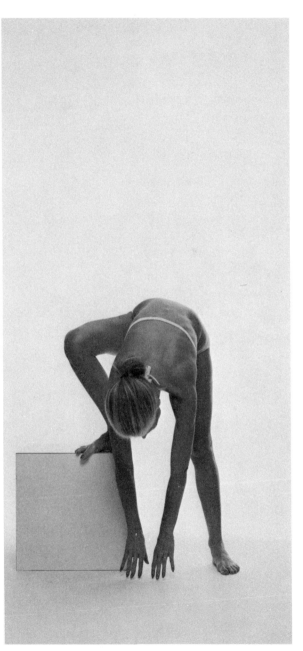

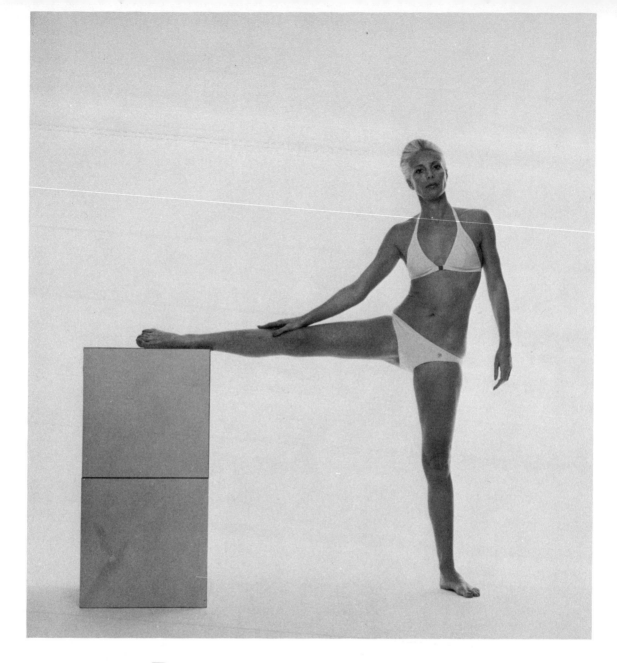

Barre and Bottom Up

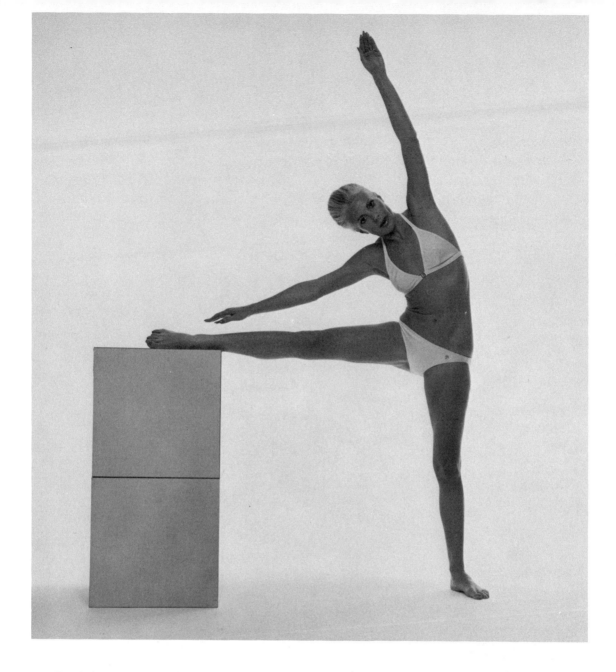

Pavlova I am not. Forget proper turnout, don't worry about grace. Neither of us is about to appear in *Swan Lake*.

The point is to use whatever you have at barre level for the marvelous tone it gives to the legs, the sharp yank at the waist when you stretch to the side, and the flexibility you gain swooping over to touch the floor.

The side stretch keeps you

from lapsing into that thick, unbendable look in the middle as if you were all of a piece from shoulders to hip: a woman in a cast.

The added grope on the floor stretches the spine and affords relief from the strain of the sideward thrust. You are getting a two-way stretch on your own body foundation.

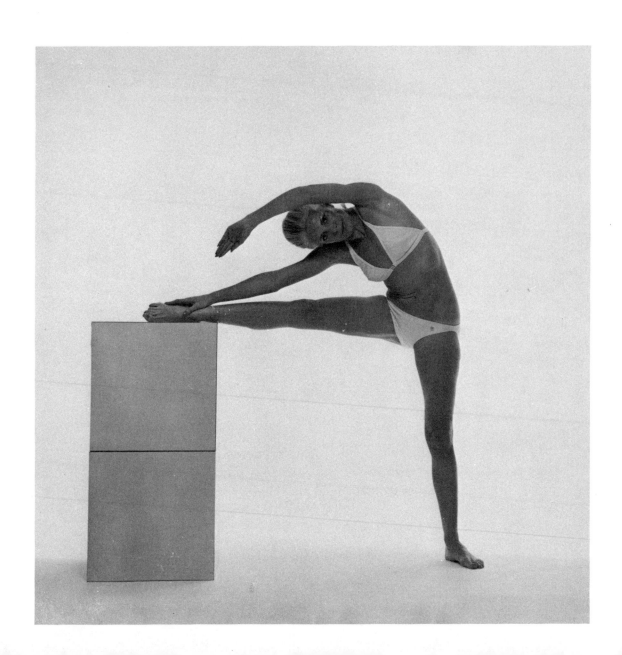

Hitch your right leg at half-mast, right arm relaxed, with hand on the knee. Both legs should be straight with knees neither bent nor locked. Raise your left arm while sliding your right hand along your right leg. As your left arm curves over as far as it can go, your right hand reaches your right ankle.

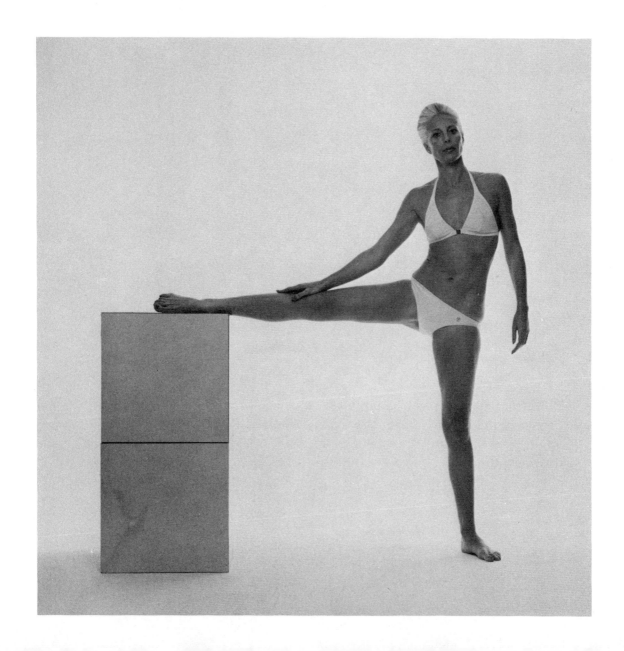

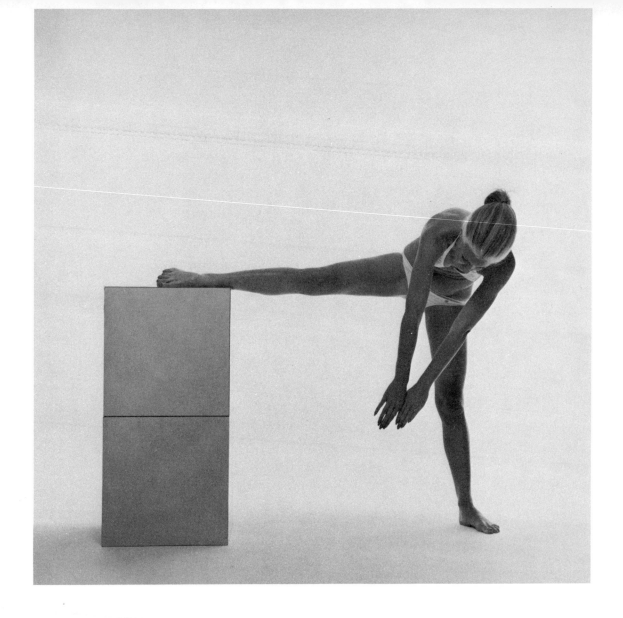

You cannot stretch to the back or you will lose your balance; and you should not hunch forward. Look to the front and swing to the side.

Swing back to beginning stance. Tuck head under lowering arms and reach for the floor on the bias. Touch there (not shown) for the extra adjustment it takes

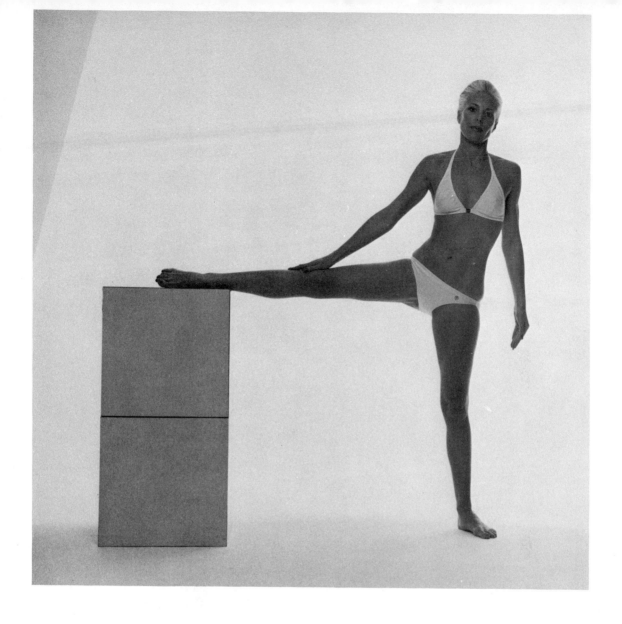

so that your right fingers touch as well. Shift to the left and scrape the floor again. You are like an old-fashioned chicken who has to scratch for its sustenance instead of being force-fed.

Raise, and repeat 20 times. Switch sides, repeat in reverse.

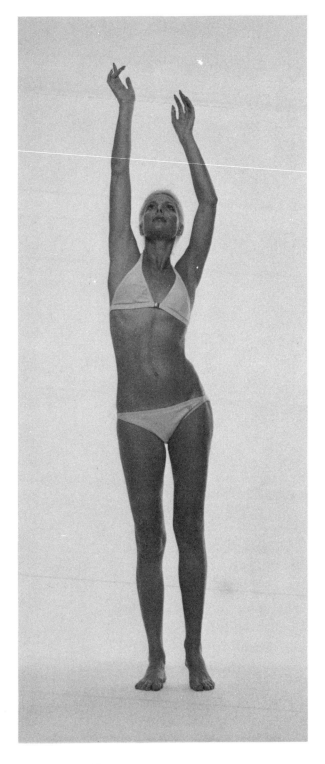
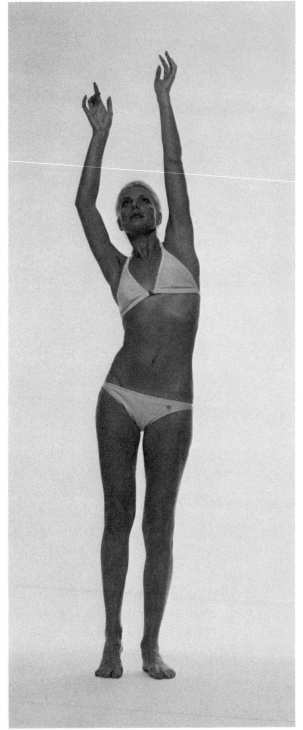

142

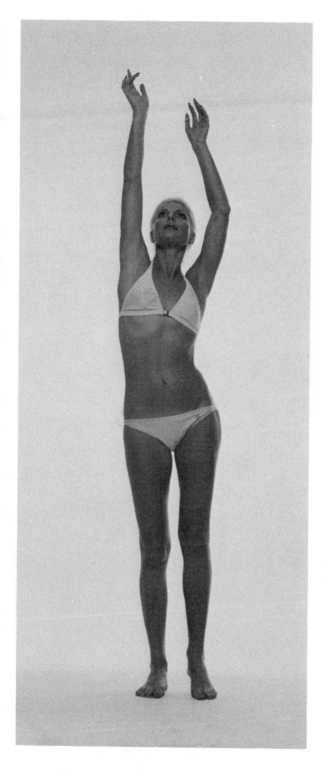

Sky-scraping

This is the classic rise-and-shine exercise. Reach for the new day. Time to get moving. Think tall.

Inhale and stretch your right arm as high as it will go. Shift at the hip—you are as thin as a greyhound through the middle— and stretch your left arm up to the clouds. Exhale. Shift at the hip. Stretch your right arm. . . .

The only thing I reach for in the morning is a hot cup of tea. I may be a "morning person," but I'm not about to exert myself unduly. I love the feel of this stretch when I am tense or have been sitting too long. As I shift from side to side, I can hear my spine crackle, sense it pull out and readjust.

For me the need for this stretch comes later in the day. At most, when I first wake up, I stretch horizontally—extremities, are you with me? For your morning alert, see the exercises that follow.

143

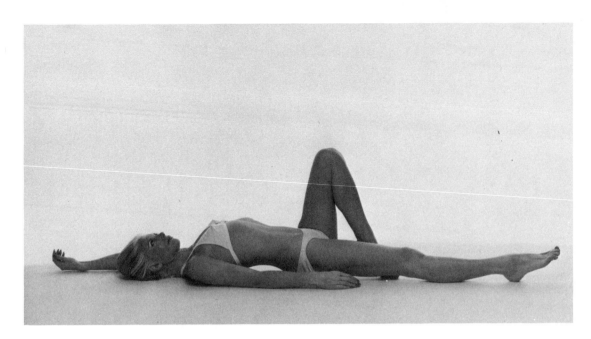

Morning
Wake Up

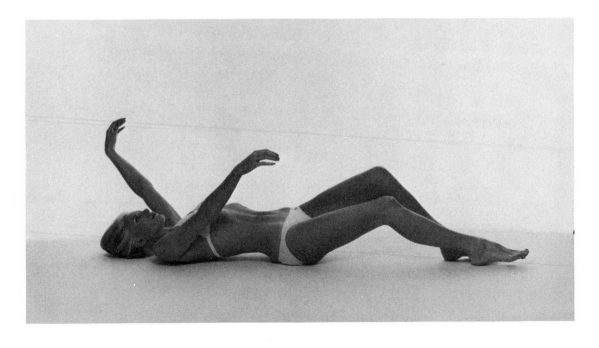

The alarm has gone off. Instead of leaping out of bed (you might have a heart attack), start with an activity so lazy it seems involuntary.

Raise your left knee and toss your left arm to the back of your head (on the pillow). Reach with left arm as far back as possible. Meanwhile stretch your flat-out right leg to the foot of the bed. It won't go that far, but that is what you think you are aiming for.

Your right arm, rather than lying inert at your right side, is also trying to grow.

Alternate arm and leg positions. Repeat, in alternation, 8 or 10 times.

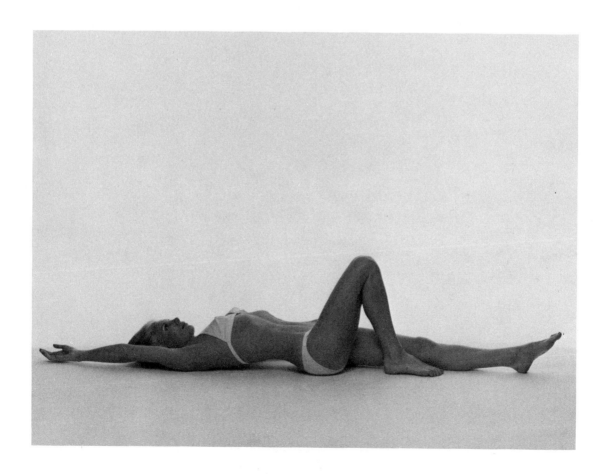

Ankles Alert

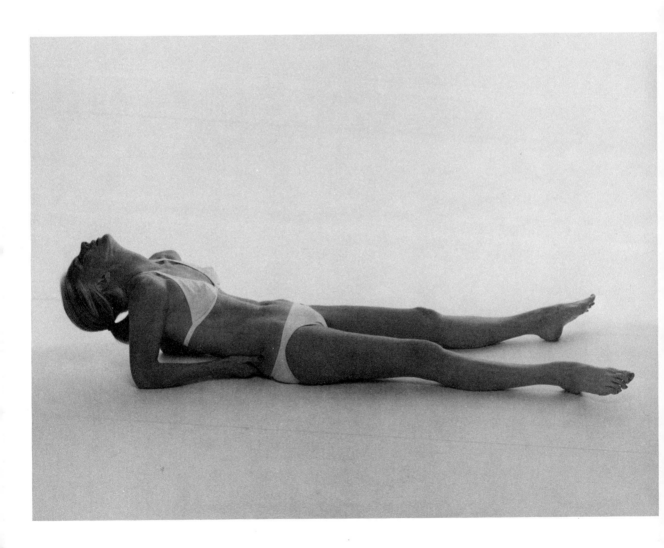

The funny thing about stretch exercise is that, depending on your mood, it either relaxes and puts you to sleep or starts up your motor again. For example, if you work out before going to bed, this is a good finale. Already horizontal, you pull out the knots at both ends and doze off.

On the other hand, the same exercise gets you going in the morning, which is when I do it. I may be wide awake, but I am not sure my body has got the message. Still in bed, I prop myself up on my elbows, arch my head back, extend my legs, and point my toes.

With torso propped—that will wake up your stomach muscles

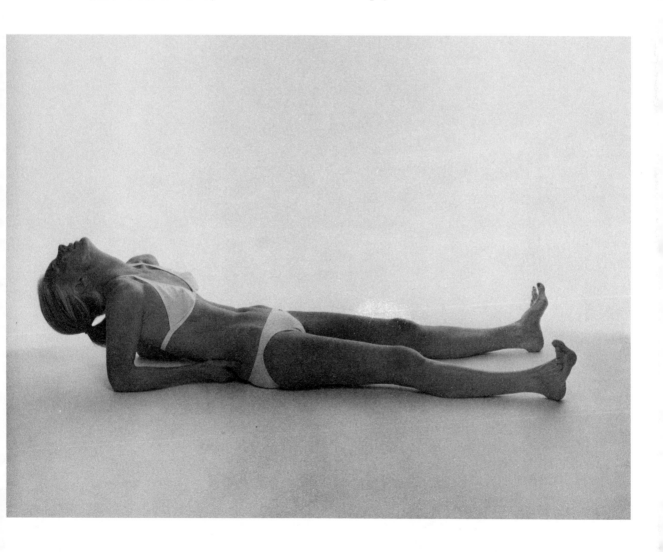

too—raise your feet perpendicularly as far as the ankles allow. Lower one foot, pointing toes. Repeat, alternating four times. Don't be namby-pamby; make those ankles work.

Return to relaxed lying position, arms at sides. Then start the sequence again: raise torso, extend legs, and so on. Repeat entire sequence 10 times.

Variations include lowering feet from the perpendicular to the side instead of forward. Or you can do circles, first to the right, then to the left.

Note: if any exertion in the

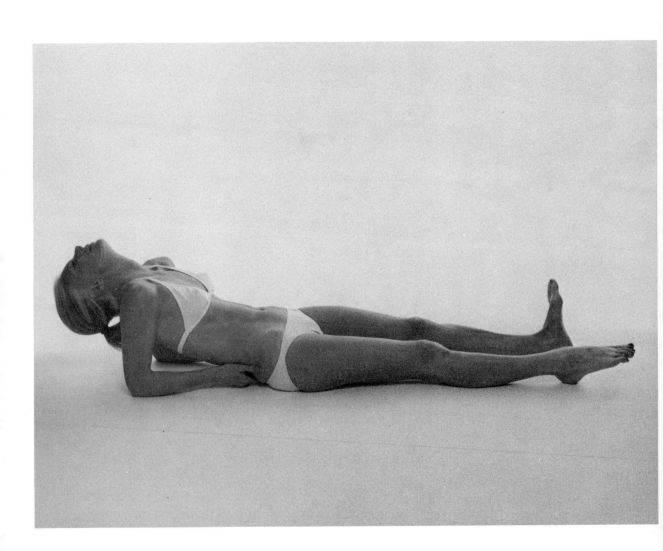

morning seems like running the last mile, there is still one motion you can make.

Stay warm and sprawled under the covers. Slowly begin to massage the sole and arch of one foot with the toes and sole of the other. As you massage, the arch begins to tingle from the friction and generate its own special heat.

Switch over and use the first pampered foot to service its mate. Get the second arch tingling. Switch back and forth once again. It may sound silly, but somehow it works—magically, physically, you want to be up on your feet, are ready to get out of bed.

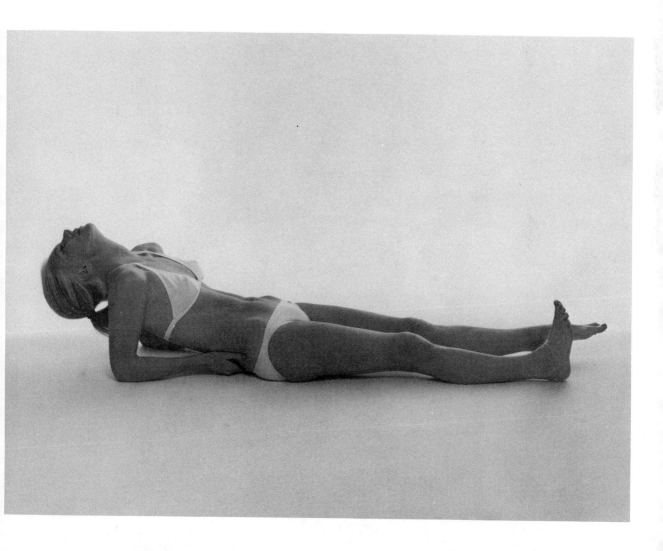

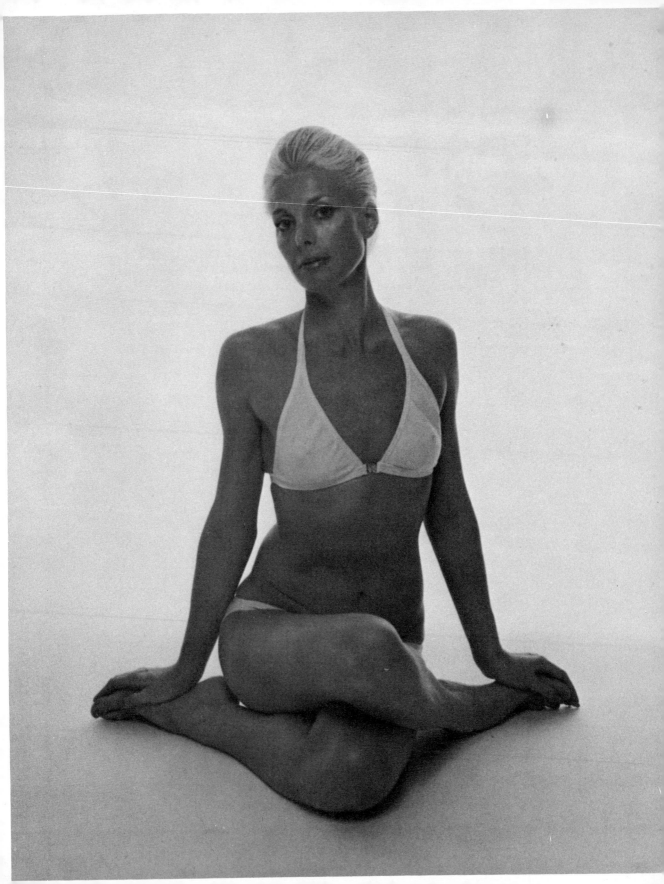

Three for TV

Assuming you aren't always watching TV in bed as a cure
for insomnia, I advise the following trio during commercial
breaks. Your thighs, hips, backside, and neck will get
the message.

I believe in sitting on the floor; it makes you more aware
of your body, and if nothing else, by getting down to floor
level and back on your feet, you exert a few muscles.

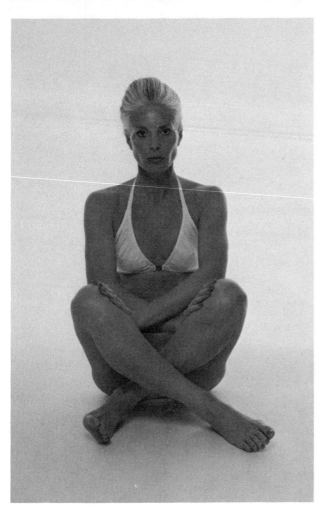 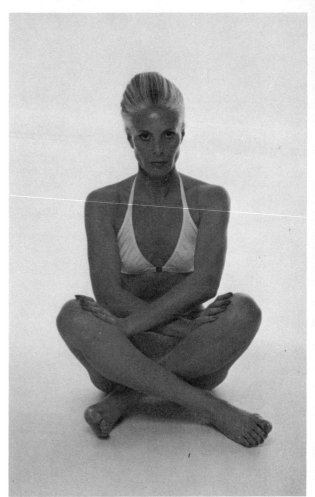

Cross
Purposes

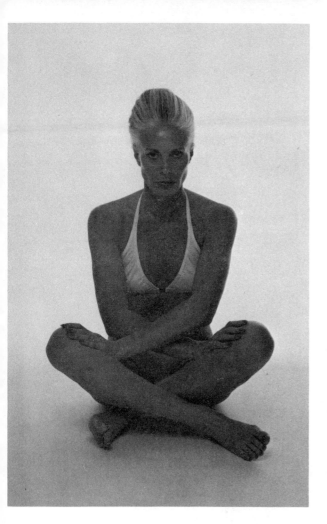
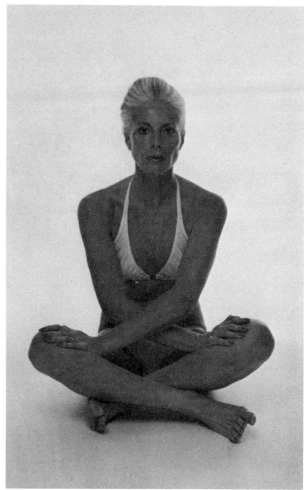

Isometrically yours, the first
exercise is for the inner thighs.
Sit cross-legged and cross-armed,
with knees at waist level. Push
with your palms against your
knees. Eventually your palms
should win, and your knees
almost flatten to the floor, but not
without resistance. That is the
key.

I don't expect your knees to go
flat out—if they can, as in yoga,
skip this isometric; your inner
thigh is vibrant enough. My legs
don't meet yoga specifications,
but they pass beauty muster,
which is my aim.

Whatever maximum span you
reach, use your palms with equal
force to stop your legs returning
to initial position. This time the
legs "win."

153

The Floor Wiper

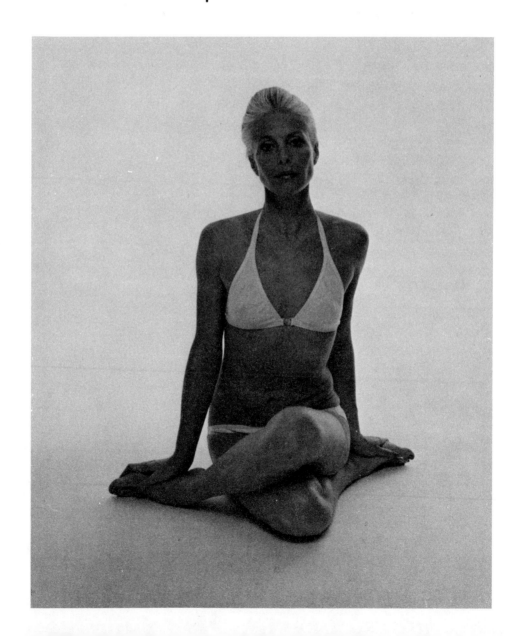

For limbering the legs and tightening buttocks and under-thigh, sit with one leg wrapped over the other. Reverse legs. Repeat 20 times. The unscrambling is easy. To reposition, haul in one or both legs by the ankles, right hand for left ankle, left hand for right ankle. Done fast it is more fun, but remember each time you rewrap to straighten your spine.

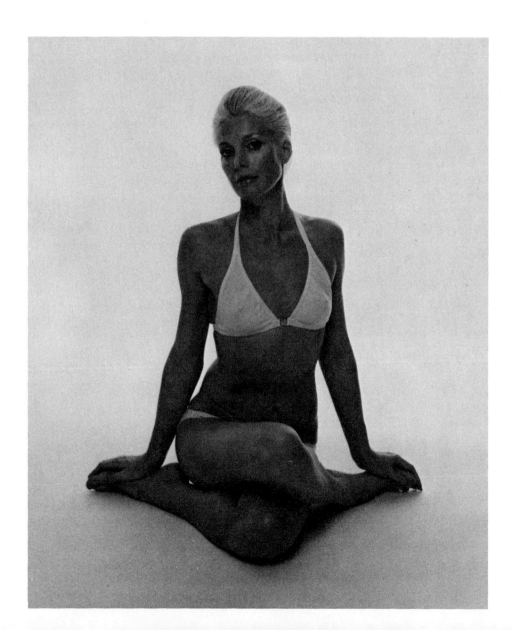

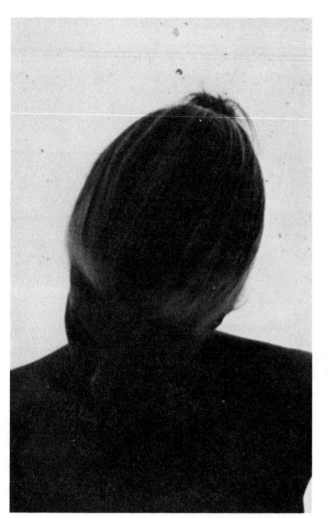
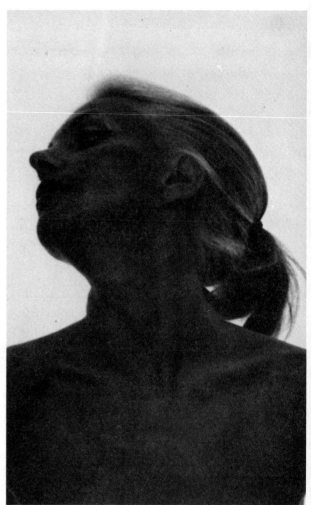

Neck Rolls

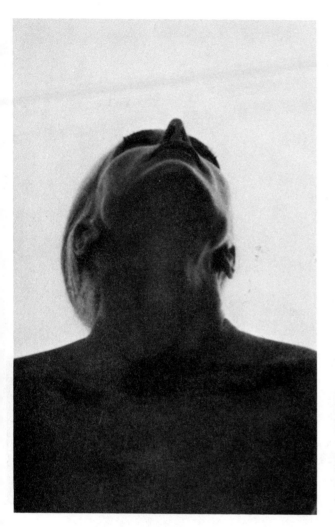
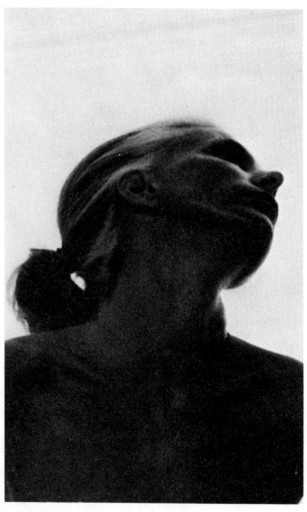

Anyone who suffers from tension in the shoulders and the back of the neck should make neck rolls a habit. You squeak and you creak and say "Aaah" with delight as you feel the tightness yield. Usually, at one point—and not always the same one—in the arc you meet with the most resistant knot. Dwell on it briefly before moving on; reach up with a hand and knead the muscle. Each time you reach full circle, swing the head around in the opposite direction. To do this 10 times is enough; you want to be loose, not dangling.

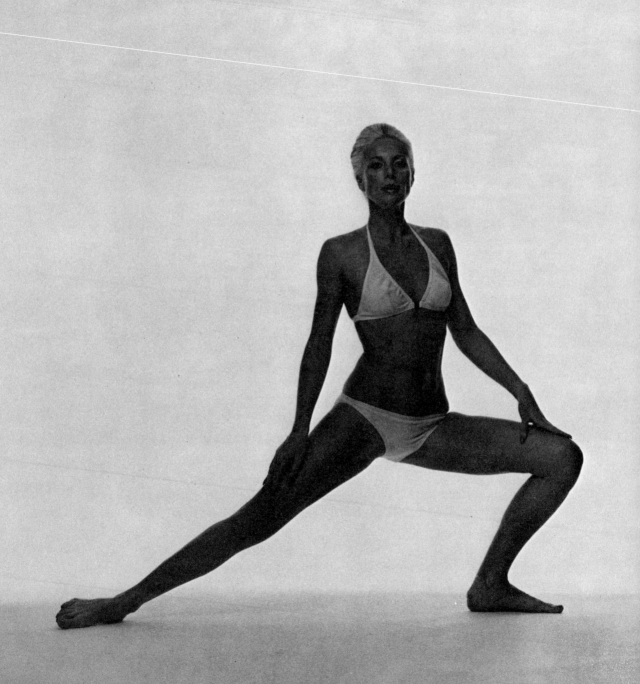

Eat Well, Eat Less

My exercises are selective. So is the way I eat. There's no sense working to keep beauty muscles alive and then tucking food away like a vacuum cleaner—or starving yourself, just to be thin.

Unless you provide your body with the proper nutrients, no one will notice the elegant line of your thighs, but will be concerned about how awful you look: a drawn or pasty face, a mottled or pale complexion.

If you're on a drastic diet, you won't have the energy to exercise. Women and men who are obsessed with staying thin—the current beauty canon—sometimes go off the deep end into fads, cults, or austerity diets: whole-grain cereals, grapefruit, high-protein jags, the honey plunge, or raw-is-good-for-you.

The faddists, however, may not be the worst off. Give and take a few people who die in their narrow tracks, most come to their senses before it is too late and go off their deprivation regimen. Being on a diet that is balanced but inadequate in quantity is more dangerous in the long run. In that case there are no early warning signals—you just shrivel. No one can fault you on what you are eating: it is always the right thing, except that it is not enough. That's like having perfect sex, but only once a month.

Basically, though, willful, compulsive undereating is the province of ascetics, a minority breed of neurotics (including teen-agers) and the rich. Indiscriminate eating is a far more common disease. Why else would 80 million Americans be overweight?

The problem is that, as much as we love to be in shape, we loathe the conflict it involves, the need to give up one pleasure for another: chocolate for contour, popcorn today for a better figure tomorrow. Eating and drinking are fun, and much of our social life centers on these activities.

Needless to say, the more girth you acquire, the less active you become. If you cannot see your toes, much less touch them, exercise becomes a weight-lifting ordeal rather than a streamlining technique. So does just plain living. It is as if you put on every morning a rucksack weighing twenty . . . fifty . . . eighty pounds under strict orders to carry it all day: remember your load is built in, not just hoisted on your back. Who wants to tote that bale of fat?

I haven't gained or lost more than six pounds in the last fifteen years, so I must have hit on something. I love to eat, and unlike some lucky people I put on weight easily—or would, were I not selective about food. I don't go on and off diets; my approach, though flexible, is long-term. Call it a permanent affliction, except I don't consider it one.

In my experience, it is harder to stick to exercise than to stop stuffing yourself. Regular exercise is deferred pleasure, a chore you do for the results. Eating, even reasonably, provides instant gratification. I don't deprive myself to maintain my proper weight. Rigid deprivation diets, except as quick starters for the very obese, never work because you feel so miserable that you cannot wait to get back to all the bad habits that made you fat in the first place.

"It's gotten so you can't enjoy anything unless it's a grapefruit or an egg," said Shirley Wood, talent coordinator for Johnny Carson's Tonight Show. I do find grapefruit enjoyable, but I don't eat three a day or exclude all other fruit.

Nor am I hung up on health foods. I don't touch packaged, sliced white bread, but neither does anyone with a taste bud left. Some of my best friends actually salivate at the prospect of yogurt and powdered yeast for breakfast. Not I. (In New York, where they are readily available, I do buy so-called natural health foods—good honey, for example— but I am not addicted. I travel too much to get hooked on anything so special that it, too, has to be remembered and packed.)

Do I have a magic solution? Cider vinegar? Brown rice? Ten glasses of water a day? No salt? No sugar? Ketosis? Self-hypnotism? Horse meat?

I don't think there is one answer: you are your own best dietician. Fat is like the common cold; it's not lethal, though it can lead to severe complications, and thus far no one knows how to prevent or cure it. There are rules and almost as many exceptions. Take two people of the same age,

161

height, occupation, and eating habits: one will stay thin, have a normal blood pressure, low cholesterol, perfect triglycerides, a happy liver . . . and the other will look a mess and be his or her doctor's despair. Maybe I exaggerate; nevertheless, people react differently to foods and dispose of calories in varying ways.

It seems to me that first you learn the basics of nutrition —and the earlier the better—and then you adjust them to personal desires and needs. For the benefit of anyone who has spent the last fifty years on a desert island, the basics are briefly as follows:

1. In order to ensure an adequate supply of the carbohydrates, fats, proteins, minerals, and vitamins your body needs, your diet should include:

    A. Whole-grain breads and cereals, also fruit (because of its natural sugar), for carbohydrates.
    B. Vegetable oils—corn, cottonseed, olive, safflower, soybean, or sunflower—as the primary source of fats.
    C. Fish, meat, poultry, eggs (and soybeans) for complete protein.
    D. Dairy products, eggs, fish, fruit, poultry, vegetables, and whole grains for mineral supply. Liver, for example, is high in iron; dairy products give you calcium; and dried beans, peas, lentils, and bananas are rich in potassium.
    E. Dairy products, eggs, fruit, organ meats, vegetables, and whole grains for vitamins.

2. Calories do count, but rather than memorize charts or carry a pocket computer, the point is to grasp the fundamentals; fatty meats, fermented cheeses, food cooked

in sauce, most highly processed foods, starches, and sweets are more fattening per average portion than lean meat and salad; avocados and bananas, for example, are richer than apples and oranges; peas and corn more than peppers, salad greens, and tomatoes; a glass of dry wine or a straight scotch has fewer calories than a beer or Coke; skim-milk cheeses and yogurt have fewer calories than homogenized milk or cream; the sugar you put in coffee or tea adds up.

If you are obese—fifty pounds or more overweight—I doubt that my system will work, because your appestat (which regulates your appetite) is probably out of whack. You eat when you are not hungry, don't know when to stop, and need controlled food therapy before you can cope by yourself. It would be like handing my exercise program to someone who has both arms and legs in a cast and has just recovered from pneumonia.

Eventually my ideas are applicable, but first get yourself to a fat farm or a strict Big Brother doctor and follow the prescribed regimen until the worst of the bulk is gone. You need medical surveillance because that amount of fat usually overlies other physical problems. As for the emotional wrench—if you can't resort to food for solace, where do you go?—let us hope you have an understanding family or friends. Perhaps, along with your blood type, credit cards, and driver's license, you should carry a small warning sign: Beware, Dieting!

My program is useful either for maintenance of proper weight or for those with a five-, ten-, or twenty-pound overweight problem who do not need rigid diets. At that level, informed common sense and a minimum of discipline that becomes a habit will keep you in line. It may take longer to lose the extra fat, but the point is to keep it off, once lost, rather than going back and forth like a Yo-Yo. Playing Yo-Yo tears your insides apart while leaving stretch marks on the surface.

To stay in shape you don't have to starve or spend your life in a gym, but you do have to watch what you eat and put your muscles to work. In both cases, tackle the big problems first: the abdominal, gluteal, and thigh muscles when it comes to exercise, the carbohydrates and fats when it comes to food.

The Selective Diet

1. *Carbohydrates, especially sweets, are the enemy.* Needless to say, they are also soothing and psychologically satisfying. If for no other reason, they are indispensable. The question is which ones and how many.

How many is precious little compared to other, more indispensable substances. If you have a sweet tooth, it has probably been capped like mine—sugar wreaks havoc on teeth—but the point is to cap the craving as well. Do not eat sweets every day and don't keep them around the house. If you drink coffee, learn to drink it without sugar, and if it tastes strange at first, switch brands to fool yourself until you realize that the coffee is your kick, not the sugar.

Unless you are one of the lucky few who prefer sour or hot, and whose idea of bliss is biting into dill pickles, red pepper, or ginger root, at first it is going to be tough. You'll have withdrawal symptoms for several weeks, after which, surprisingly enough, you will be able to take or leave sweets. Mostly you leave sweets, because by the simple, radical act of cutting out danish pastries and desserts, chocolate, ice cream, or whatever jam you are into, you open up a large range of permissible foods.

The other carbohydrate glut to eliminate is overprocessed convenience products, whether canned, frozen, bottled, or packaged. (I do not refer to items such as canned tuna or frozen fish or shellfish, plain fruits or vegetables that can be salvaged by decent cooking, or the classic condiments.) It is the instant dinner or instant dressing that has to go. Almost all contain hidden sugar and sludge that accumulates in the body, providing what are known as "empty" calories—and full backsides. Stop buying them. Use fresh foods and make your own sauces. If you want to stay thin, you won't want many of the latter, anyway.

On the other hand, what is the one fattening, starchy, unsweet staple you eat with great pleasure? Bread? Cornmeal? Kasha? Pasta? Potatoes? Rice? Eat it! Don't take seconds, and when trying to lose weight cut to half portions, but keep the habit. It's your security blanket. My weakness is pasta, beautiful, unredeemed carbohydrate (the enriched stuff is terrible). I have it four to five times a week and always with sauce.

Sometimes I have a baked potato instead, scooped and stuffed with sour cream and minced dried beef, or just with lots of margarine. One day I might have crêpes for a change . . . it doesn't sound like dieting, does it? Most dieting does not take account of the sensual as well as the nutritional satisfaction of certain foods—as if we had no eyes or nose or palate. These diets ignore all emotional ties toward food and even make what is good for us (eggs, fish, meat, vegetables, and so on) unpalatable by insisting they always be served plain.

I have started with carbohydrates on purpose, for, as the classic forbidden fruit of dieting, they best illustrate my approach. Remember, you are looking for a permanent route to weight stabilization, and because of this, you are willing to be selective. Rather than "uppers" of random eating interspersed with "downers" of deprivation, the aim is to find your balance.

Because I get the pasta I enjoy, I don't eat:

A. Other starches: toast or bread (except as a "pusher"), cereal, rice, pancakes, or pizza.
B. Snacks.
C. Sugar (I put honey in my tea).
D. Desserts, except for cheese and/or fruit.

I do pop a chocolate now and again, perhaps twice a week, as a reward to myself for being good. If you are carbohydrate-frugal on a day-to-day basis, the occasional chocolate does not spell doom to weight maintenance— abstain only when trying to lose.

In fact, though it is diet heresy, were my sweet tooth truly compulsive I would have my favorite dessert four or five times a week, allowing for it by cutting out starches during the first and second courses. Pasta may not be ideal—from a nutritional point of view, I'd be better off with whole-wheat bread—but I believe that you should think thin on your own terms. Make the decisions you can keep over the long haul, so that diet and pleasure are not antagonistic.

2. *Fats are the other villain in most diet schemes.* Whether for losing weight or lowering cholesterol levels, butter is taboo, lard and olive oil unthinkable, and you are supposed to eat vegetables and salad with a squeeze of

lemon, salt, and pepper—or totally unadorned. That will put you off them for life!

When a recipe calls for butter, I substitute margarine, though it may be unnecessary, considering the small amounts of fat involved. Still, I so rarely eat creamed food or gravies —and that is the essential decision—that if once in a while I choose a béarnaise, béchamel, or hollandaise sause, then I do it without guilt.

A certain amount of lubricant is necessary; it is the overdose that is to be avoided.

3. *Proteins, minerals, and vitamins are friends.* I put no limitation on the amount of cheese, eggs, meat, fish, fruit, and raw or cooked vegetables I eat, except to balance flavors and textures; my preoccupation is more gourmet than dietetic. I don't go in for jumbo steaks and thick slabs of meat because I find it more interesting to have several courses and variety. You cannot stay in shape and have muscle without protein, but unless you lead a very active outdoors life, you don't need a tiger's kill. Too much meat, like too much of anything, makes you fat or deprives you of room for other equally valuable food. Man does not live by meat alone.

When it comes to fruits and vegetables, the reason for eating them fresh and in season is gourmet, as well as nutritional. Apart from the difference in enzymes, vitamins, and minerals, a winter tomato is flat while a summer tomato with basil is divine. It may be fun in the grand manner to have perishables in midwinter. I prefer to let the seasons take their course: why should January taste like June?

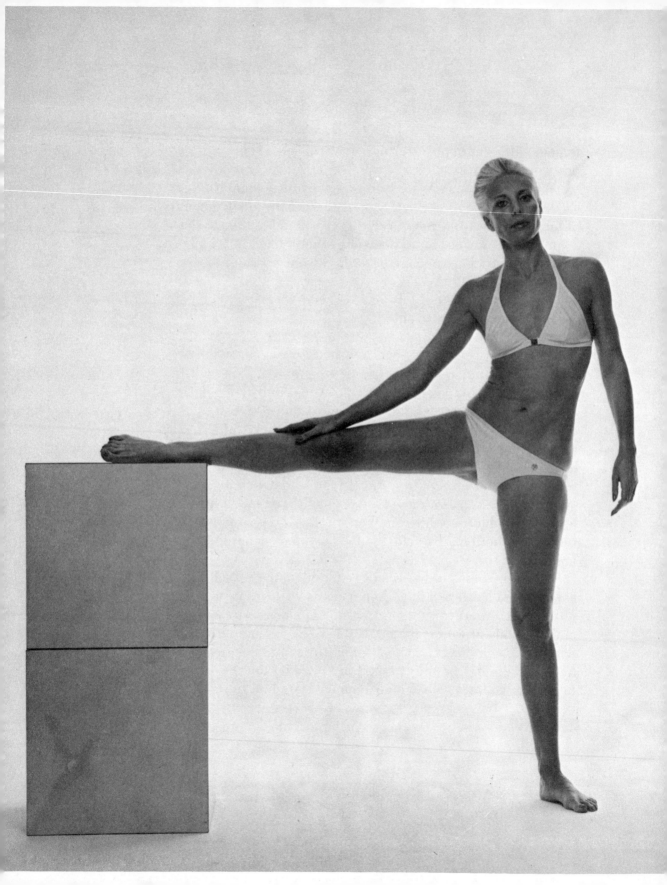

Answering Your Questions on Diets

What about Snacks?

Cut them out. Is life so dull you have to keep munching all
the time? If it is anxiety you are feeding, try worry beads or
therapy, or take up knitting.

The usual suggestion is to eat a piece of fruit—people
have been known to eat the core, and you are supposed to
keep carrot sticks on the ready. They don't satisfy and never
will; the only real solution is to put snacking itself out of
mind. Eating well at mealtimes, when you are supposed to
eat, helps a great deal. Snacking often stems from such

indifferent cooking that you get up from the table-overstuffed but underfed.

As usual, there are exceptions, such as the case of a person whose metabolism (or ulcer) is such that he/she is much better off with frequent small meals rather than three regulation feedings. You are not snacking but dividing normal intake by five or six instead of three. Most work schedules make this difficult, but if you have to, you learn to pack and carry your emergency brown bag.

Do You Recommend Low-Calorie Drinks?

The best one is water. Straight from the tap or fountain, home-bottled and chilled if you prefer, mineral water if the local brew is polluted. I drink it plain or with a squirt of lemon.

When you are thirsty and do not know what you want— beer, ginger ale, Coke, orangeade—the best answer is water. But it never occurs to you, strangely enough: one has to be reconditioned to the obvious.

The only time I would ban water is before ordering a meal. Unless it is gingerly sipped, water tends to make you feel bloated if drunk with meals.

I also don't recommend slugging it down when you are overheated from exercise or the sun. Again, either sip or, if circumstances permit, swish it around in your mouth and spit it out. That takes away the parched sensation without shocking the system. You can have more when you are calm, cool, and collected. Often the more you drink when it is hot, the thirstier and the more uncomfortable you become.

Under less climatic stress, have all the water between meals you want. Drinking water does not cause fat due to water retention. Salt does that, whereas water helps you get rid of toxins.

Coffee and tea, without honey, milk, or sugar, are also low-calorie, but they are stimulants. You probably know yourself well enough to judge how much you can take without getting jittery. If tea revs you up, try substituting an herbal tea or infusion—rose hip, for example, is rich in vitamin C, camomile soothes and has mild laxative properties.

How Much Meat or Fish Do I Need for Body-Building and Muscle Tone?

I get by on meat (including chicken) twice a week and fish several times a week. You may need more or less. Some people thrive on meat and eat it three times a day. This would knock me out, but the point I keep stressing is that we are not all alike.

One exception to the rule is when I'm traveling around the country. Then the only safe haven seems to be meat— steak without sauces.

Usually the first thing I look for on entering the hotel room is the "fridge" where I can store a few items from the local grocer like papaya, peaches, yogurt—then it's meat at noon, fruit for dinner, and early to bed in the evening . . . I trot off to sleep feeling purified.

Beyond a certain point, eating meat does not help put on more muscle, and the only justification for demanding it is psychological. Many of us are so conditioned that a meal without meat leaves us frustrated. We get up from the table feeling we really have not eaten: Oh! for a good thick, juicy steak! If meat gives you satisfaction, then make it a prominent, permanent part of your own selective diet. But do not become so programmed that you fear your performance will suffer unless you get it—that is a myth like the "Breakfast of Champions."

What about a Vegetarian Diet?

I feel listless without meat or fish. However, there are surely many vegetarians with beautiful bodies and more pep than I. My hunch is that they are "natural" vegetarians who have gravitated toward an eating style because of their dislike of the taste, texture, and smell of meat.

As long as you eat eggs and sufficient dairy products (milk, yogurt, white cheeses), or have a passion for soybeans, you will probably get enough protein. Vegetarians as a rule are also health-conscious, and they use wheat germ and yeast supplements, both of which boost the protein ration, as well as being high in minerals and vitamins.

The mistake is to depend solely on legumes and nuts, because their protein ration is incomplete, unless balanced with whole grains. That is when you begin to dwell on the spiritual side of things, for you don't have the physical energy to do otherwise.

Do Seasonings Affect the Look of Your Body?

I have never looked at a person and instantly surmised, "This one's a pepper girl." However, too much salt is easy to spot. It shows up in cellulite bulges and bumps or rapid ups and downs of weight due to fluctuating water retention and loss.

Take it easy with the salt shaker. You don't have to touch it at table—if you seasoned enough while cooking. If you catch yourself starting to sprinkle salt on your food before even tasting it (a bad habit), salt your palm instead; gather the salt up with the fingers of your other hand and throw the pinch over your shoulder for good luck. Better gritty floors than bumpy thighs!

When I first trained myself to cut back on salt, I read a table of food composition as a quick refresher course. In many instances, you can rely on your taste buds; a soft- or hard-boiled egg improves with a dash of salt, but bacon or ham and eggs rarely need it because the meat is salty already. Nonetheless, one is apt to forget the hidden salt in butter and margarine, to say nothing of most condiments, such as garlic salt and bottled sauces. Finally I discovered diet salt.

The only season to throw caution to the winds is summertime, when it is so hot and muggy, the perspiration beads on the forehead and drips down your nose, and you would like to take twelve showers a day. Don't worry then about water-retention fat—you are sweating it off and need the salt to avoid dehydration.

Why Are You Supposed to Eat a Big Breakfast?

After ten or more hours of abstinence, you need food to get you going again, and if you start off well fueled, you won't be so hungry that you stuff yourself at lunch and spend most of the afternoon in a daze.

Physiologically, a sturdy breakfast makes sense. Once again, however, it all depends on the individual. I cannot face food when I first get up—all I want is grapefruit and tea. I don't get the eleven o'clock empties; in fact, mornings are the best time for me. So why eat? I feel fine without it.

The basic rule for maintaining proper weight is:

EAT ONLY WHEN YOU ARE HUNGRY.

Trust your appetite unless it is wildly out of whack, and the quickest way to throw it out is to feel obliged to eat whether or not you're hungry.

If you wake up hungry or feel that way midmorning, it is equally foolish to try and get by on black coffee. Reach for fruit and protein foods (eggs, cheese, milk, yogurt, bacon, ham—even a hamburger) and keep carbohydrates to a minimum, especially cereals and sweet rolls. These often trigger the appetite rather than satisfying it. If you long for toast, have it. Then for lunch, do not eat a sandwich but have soup or a salad and no bread.

Does Drinking Affect Body Tone and Is It Fattening?

If you are a bottle-a-day girl, you may wind up with the build of Winston Churchill, though not be blessed with the brains.

The classic beer belly is hard to lose by exercise alone. Furthermore, heavy drinking tends to thicken the middle (double the number of abdominal exercises and cut consumption by half). It also encourages cellulite, puffiness, double chins, jowls, and dry, crepey skin. Moderate drinking does not necessarily make you fat. There are even advanced alcoholics who are thin, but that is because they have lost all interest in food, not a solution I would recommend.

I rarely touch alcohol for the simple reason that it makes me look and feel liverish. A little wine with meals, a split of champagne, a shot of hard liquor twenty times a year (usually to give me courage to make a promotion speech). . . .

On the other hand, I don't expect everyone to be so abstemious. A certain amount of alcohol is said to increase longevity. If drinking is part of your day, and your metabolism burns it up without bloat and hangover headache, go ahead and indulge. You know best what you can handle, and as with all cravings, you compensate by being strict in other areas.

1. Were I to drink, I would make sure my diet was super-rich in the vitamin B's.

2. I would drink hard or soft liquor dry and straight, or on the rocks. That is what most connoisseur drinkers do, and their instincts are right. Sweet wines and liqueurs are higher in calories. So are barmen's specials and highballs, because

of the ginger ale, tonic water, or cola that is added to the alcohol. Forget beer if you want to stay trim.

3. Have your alcohol buzz, but don't blur the issue by munching while you are at it. This doesn't include having wine with meals, which is a civilized habit. It is the cocktail munch that has to go: the salted nuts, olives, canapés, and dips. They load you with sodium and calories and wreck your appetite for a balanced meal.

4. If you drink, restrict your intake of sugary carbohydrates. In fact, a lot of drinkers who suddenly go on the wagon discover a sweet tooth they never had so long as they got their alcohol.

5. Exercise, take walks, be active—the more toxins you absorb, the more you need to work off.

Does Smoking Help Keep You Trim?

The only way to stay thin is to discover by trial and error how much and what you can eat and make it a habit. Putting on weight after giving up smoking is a common complaint because people substitute food for tobacco to satisfy an oral compulsion. On the other hand, many smokers will assure you that smoking opens up their appetite rather than depressing it.

There have been so many reports on how detrimental heavy smoking is to health, I need add no further warning. My solution is to enjoy a half-dozen thin cigars a day, using them as a reward for plowing through a hard job or the usual boring tasks that have to be performed to keep the ship afloat.

If you feel you must smoke:

1. Make sure you have a balanced diet rich in Vitamin C and all the B's. In other words, compensate for your favorite poison.

2. Pull in all the oxygen you can; check that you are breathing correctly and arrange your work schedule to include regular blasts of fresh air. After years of smoking you are no longer an ace at tennis or underwater swimming, but my mild program should not set off a coughing fit—and at least, while exercising you won't be lighting up.

Does It Matter When I Have My Biggest Meal?

How you distribute food over the course of the day is strictly individual. I have a light breakfast and supper; my heaviest (in carbohydrates) meal is lunch, preceded by a light breakfast. This gives me the push to get through an active afternoon. Then, unless I'm entertaining or going out, my program is a quiet dinner and early to bed. When faced with a series of social dinners, I switch to a light meal at noon.

What counts is the total intake of calories, not their timing. It is better to eat at regular intervals than to skip now, gorge later, so your stomach and belly are not worked like an accordion with all the resultant swelling and pleats.

Were I a night owl, dinner would be my big meal because, getting up late, I would not want much lunch.

Find the pattern that suits you best with occasional and seasonal variations: big lunches on very hot days make you sleepy unless you are air-conditioned (hence the siesta).

Must I Broil Meat to Stay Thin?

The broiling of (lean) meat is recommended in most diets because it limits intake of animal fat = calories + cholesterol. The obsession with fat may be on the wane because it now appears that sugar rather than fat is the real cholesterol bugaboo. I like lean meat, but it is expensive, and pretty boring unless you sauce it up. Broiled calves' liver, for example, not only has to be sliced thicker, it still tastes like leather and cannot compare with thinner slices quickly sautéed. Butter, wine, herbs, and pepper help.

It is a good habit to cut off the fat and leave it on the side of your plate (most children do this instinctively), but that does not mean you cannot use lamb, mutton, pork, or cheaper cuts of beef and veal in the kitchen. Bacon lends itself to broiling, but draining it on paper towels eliminates excess grease. Of course, you should go light on breaded fried cutlets and chicken or at least be aware when you eat them, as I do, that you compensate by omitting other fried foods the next day.

Roasts, stews, casseroles, and boiled meat have more calories than broiled lean veal steak, but none of this sturdy fare is going to make you fat. It is the junk food and the compulsive snacking all day long that do so.

What About Condiments and Ready-Made Dressings and Sauces?

As a rule, make your own dressings and sauces—they taste better and at least you know what is in them. If you have twenty pounds or more to lose, cream sauces and gravies are an obvious taboo, and chances are you will discover they were smothering flavor instead of adding to it. Conversely, the habit of reaching for ketchup, mustard, or relish often stems from an understandable attempt to give some zest to bland institutional food.

I would never eliminate ready-made condiments entirely —certain excellent dishes for weight-conscious people cry out for soy sauce, Worcestershire, Tabasco, or mustard, and most of us get an occasional craving for less classic stuff—instant avocado sauce mix, for instance, is a marvel of chemistry with a long list of ingredients that implausibly tastes the way the real fruit should. Pregnant women often get dill pickle yen. Unscientific, maybe—why should pickles stave off discomfort and nausea? But illusion or not, it sure beats recourse to pharmaceuticals.

You have to allow for a few predilections, even fanciful ones, in an otherwise sober routine. The point is to be aware that you are either adding "empty" calories or sharply increasing your intake of salt. If part of your weight problem is excess water retention, be sparing with condiments. With that exception, a penchant for sharp, hot, and sour tastes as opposed to sweet is a lifelong blessing for proper weight maintenance.

Why the Emphasis on Salad and Raw Vegetables?

A meal without a simple or mixed salad vinaigrette seems incomplete to me. From the nutritional point of view, fresh raw salad and vegetables have more vitamins, enzymes, and minerals than do limp, overcooked ones. Does anyone, however, still overcook vegetables, or throw out most of their virtue with the water in which they have been cooked? It is so easy to steam them quickly or learn to stir-fry them in a very little oil.

Apart from the pleasure of crisp salad, which I doubt I'd forgo even if it were fattening, there are reasons for emphasizing it:

1. It's a way to wean yourself from convenience foods and restore a sensitivity to the taste of the real thing.

2. Beans have to be snapped, asparagus scrubbed, peas podded, and artichokes trimmed. Washing, slicing, or shredding raw vegetables and snipping a few fresh herbs takes hardly any time at all, as does the washing and draining of salad. Any woman who is busy but still likes to eat well believes in salads.